ESSENTIAL INTERMITTENT FASTING

THE COMPLETELY NEW GUIDE

Discover new methods on how to awaken your metabolism, lose weight effectively, and embrace enduring and harmonious well-being.

by

Giuliano Monti

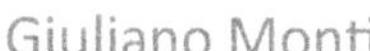

Summary

Chapter 1: Introduction to Intermittent Fasting

1.1 History and Origin of Intermittent Fasting

Intermittent fasting, a practice that alternates periods of food intake with periods of fasting, is deeply rooted in a rich and diverse history. This practice is not a modern concept but has its origins in historical epochs and cultural practices dating back thousands of years.

Since ancient times, fasting has been an intrinsic component of human societies, often intertwined with religious rites, spiritual practices, and survival necessities. In ancient cultures such as those of Greece, Rome, and India, fasting was practiced for both spiritual and physical reasons. Hippocrates, the father of modern medicine, recommended fasting as an effective means to improve health, a view shared by many other historical figures, including Plato and Aristotle.

Throughout the ages, fasting has maintained a significant role in the world's major religions. For example, Ramadan in the Islamic world, Yom Kippur in Judaism, and Lent in Christianity are all examples of periods during which the faithful practice forms of fasting. In these traditions, fasting is seen as an act of purification, a way to exercise self-control, and a gesture of solidarity towards the less fortunate.

The practice of intermittent fasting, as we know it today, began to take shape in the 20th century, when scientific research started to explore its health effects more deeply. One of the earliest significant studies on intermittent fasting dates back to the 1930s, when it was discovered that alternate day fasting could prolong life in rodents. This paved the way for a series of research studies that examined the various health benefits associated with intermittent fasting, such as improved metabolism and reduced risk of some chronic diseases.

In the 21st century, interest in intermittent fasting has grown exponentially, thanks to its popularity among public figures and the spread of scientific studies confirming its benefits. With the advent of social media and an increased self-awareness about health, more and more people have turned to this practice as a tool to improve their physical and mental well-being.

In this historical and cultural context, intermittent fasting is not just a passing trend, but an ancient practice with solid historical and scientific roots. Its rediscovery and popularity in modern times reflect a growing awareness of the need to return to a more natural and rhythmic approach to eating, in contrast to the continuous eating patterns that characterize modern life.

In the next section, we will explore the scientific principles behind intermittent fasting. This will allow us to better understand how this ancient practice has been rediscovered through the lens of modern science, providing a solid foundation for its use as a tool to improve health and wellness.

1.2 Basic Scientific Principles of Intermittent Fasting

After exploring the history and origins of intermittent fasting, it is essential to understand the scientific principles underlying this practice. This understanding not only strengthens our confidence in intermittent fasting as a tool for health and wellness but also helps us to implement it more effectively.

Intermittent fasting operates through several biological and biochemical mechanisms that profoundly affect our body. One of the core concepts is the transition from the fed state to the fasting state. Normally, when we eat, our body uses glucose derived from carbohydrates as the main source of energy. Excess glucose is stored as glycogen in the liver and muscles and, beyond a certain threshold, as fat in adipose tissues.

During fasting, once glycogen reserves are depleted, the body begins to burn accumulated fats to produce energy. This process, known as ketosis, is one of the key benefits of intermittent fasting, as it promotes weight loss and improves lipid metabolism.

Another fundamental aspect is the effect of intermittent fasting on cellular processes, particularly autophagy. Autophagy is a 'cellular cleaning' process, where cells degrade and recycle damaged or non-functional cellular components. During fasting, increased autophagy contributes to improved cellular health and reduces the risk of age-related diseases.

Intermittent fasting also has significant effects on hormone levels. For example, it increases insulin sensitivity, reducing the risk of type 2 diabetes. Moreover, it boosts levels of growth hormone, which has important effects on body composition, muscle growth, and overall well-being.

On the cognitive level, research has shown that intermittent fasting can have positive effects on brain health. This includes improved cognitive function, a reduced risk of neurodegenerative diseases, and a potential neuroprotective effect. These benefits are attributed to a combination of factors, including reduced inflammation and oxidative stress, and an increase in the production of neurotrophins, which support the growth and survival of neurons.

Finally, intermittent fasting positively affects the immune system and the inflammatory process. By reducing chronic inflammation, it can help prevent or manage various inflammatory and autoimmune conditions.

In conclusion, the scientific principles of intermittent fasting reveal a powerful impact on various aspects of human health, extending well beyond mere weight loss. This understanding provides us with solid ground to explore how intermittent fasting may be misunderstood or misrepresented, a topic we will address in the next section.

1.3 Popularity and Misconceptions of Intermittent Fasting

In recent years, intermittent fasting has become extremely popular as a tool for weight loss and health improvement. However, with this growing attention, numerous misconceptions have also emerged that deserve to be examined and clarified.

The popularity of intermittent fasting is partly due to its simplicity and flexibility, making it attractive to a wide variety of people. Unlike restrictive and complicated diets, intermittent fasting focuses on when to eat rather than what to eat. This approach makes it a viable option for those looking to improve their lifestyle without completely overturning their eating habits.

Despite its effectiveness and documented benefits, intermittent fasting is often surrounded by misconceptions. One of the most common is the idea that it equates to extreme deprivation or a form of anorexia. In reality, intermittent fasting is a controlled and conscious practice that encourages regular and nutritious food intake periods. It is crucial to differentiate it from unhealthy food restriction practices.

Another common misconception is that intermittent fasting is a quick fix for weight loss. While it can be an effective weight loss tool, its real value lies in promoting a healthier and more sustainable approach to eating. The weight loss achieved with intermittent fasting should be seen as part of a long-term shift towards healthier eating habits.

Furthermore, there is a mistaken belief that intermittent fasting is suitable for everyone. It is important to emphasize that, like any significant dietary change, it may not be appropriate for certain individuals, such as those with specific medical conditions, pregnant or breastfeeding women, and individuals with a history of eating disorders. It is always recommended to consult a doctor before starting any fasting regimen.

Another misconception concerns nutrition. Some believe that during the eating windows, it is possible to consume any type of food, regardless of its nutritional quality. However, to maximize the benefits of intermittent fasting, it is crucial to focus on a balanced and nutritious diet during the eating periods.

These misconceptions, if not addressed, can hinder the effectiveness and potential benefits of intermittent fasting. In the next section, we will discuss the goals and expected benefits of this practice, providing a clear and realistic picture of what can be achieved through a correct and informed approach to intermittent fasting.

1.4 Goals and Expected Benefits of Intermittent Fasting

Having explored the popularity and misconceptions surrounding intermittent fasting, it's important to define the realistic goals and benefits this practice can offer. Understanding these aspects is crucial for adopting an informed and sustainable approach to intermittent fasting.

Goals of Intermittent Fasting

The primary goals of intermittent fasting extend beyond mere weight loss. This practice aims to promote overall better health, greater control overeating, and an improvement in quality of life. A key objective is to develop a healthier relationship with food, learning to distinguish between physical and emotional hunger and responding more mindfully to the body's hunger and satiety signals.

Another important goal is to improve insulin sensitivity and optimize metabolism, thus helping to prevent and manage conditions such as type 2 diabetes. Furthermore, intermittent fasting aims to encourage a more active and mindful lifestyle, promoting greater attention to the quality of foods consumed and their preparation.

Expected Benefits of Intermittent Fasting

- **Sustainable Weight Loss** Unlike crash diets, intermittent fasting promotes gradual and sustainable weight loss. By regulating mealtimes, the body learns to use fat reserves as an energy source, leading to a reduction in body fat.

- **Improved Metabolic Health: ** Intermittent fasting can enhance various aspects of metabolic health, including better blood sugar regulation and a reduced risk of developing metabolic diseases.

- **Longevity and Disease Prevention: ** Some research suggests that intermittent fasting may contribute to a longer and healthier life by reducing inflammation and improving cellular stress resistance mechanisms, which are key factors in the aging process and disease prevention.

- **Mental and Cognitive Health: ** Intermittent fasting has been associated with mental health benefits, such as increased mental clarity and a reduced risk of neurodegenerative disorders, thanks to its positive influence on neuroplasticity and brain function.

- **Increased Energy and Overall Well-being: ** Many practitioners of intermittent fasting report higher energy levels and an overall improvement in well-being, attributed to the normalization of hormonal levels and improved metabolic efficiency.

Concluding this chapter, we will move on to an overview of the book in section 1.5, where we will summarize the key themes to be addressed in the following chapters. This will allow us to have a comprehensive view of how intermittent fasting can be integrated into daily life to achieve optimal health and lasting well-being.

1.5 Book Overview and What to Expect in the Coming Chapters

Concluding our first chapter, it's essential to provide an overview of what readers can expect in the following chapters. This book, "Natural and Rejuvenating Rhythms: The Complete Guide to Intermittent Fasting," is structured to guide the reader through every aspect of intermittent fasting, from theory to practice, emphasizing the importance of a holistic approach to well-being and health.

Next Steps on the Journey

The journey we will undertake together through this book is structured to provide not only a deep understanding of intermittent fasting but also to equip readers with the knowledge and tools necessary for effectively implementing it into their daily lives.

Chapter 2: Understanding Metabolism

Chapter 2 will delve into the concept of metabolism. This chapter is crucial for understanding how intermittent fasting affects our body at a metabolic level. We will explore the differences between basal and active metabolism and how intermittent fasting optimizes these functions to enhance health and weight loss.

Chapter 3: Various Forms of Intermittent Fasting

In Chapter 3, we will dive into the different forms of intermittent fasting. From 16/8 to 5:2, the chapter will provide a detailed overview of the various methods and advice on how to choose the one that best suits personal needs.

Chapter 4: Planning and Preparing for Fasting

Chapter 4 will focus on planning and preparation for fasting. This includes physical and mental preparation, creating a personalized fasting plan, and practical tips for integrating fasting into daily life.

Subsequent Chapters: From Weight Loss to Long-Term Benefits

In the subsequent chapters, we will delve into how intermittent fasting facilitates sustainable weight loss (Chapter 5), how to overcome challenges (Chapter 6), and explore the long-term health benefits (Chapter 7). Each chapter is designed to build on the previous, providing a comprehensive and exhaustive guide.

A Holistic Approach

In addition to exploring the scientific and practical aspects of intermittent fasting, this book will also dedicate chapters to complementary themes such as nutrition (Chapter 8) and the preparation of recipes and dietary tips (Chapter 9). This will ensure that the reader can adopt a holistic approach, understanding not only the 'how' but also the 'why' behind dietary choices during intermittent fasting.

Conclusion and Additional Resources

The book will conclude with a summary of key concepts (Chapter 10) and a list of additional resources (Chapter 11), providing the reader with further tools to continue their journey towards wellness.

This book is not just a guide to intermittent fasting but an invitation to explore and transform one's relationship with food and health. In the next chapter, we will begin this journey by delving into metabolism, a fundamental topic for fully understanding the impact and benefits of intermittent fasting.

Chapter 2: Understanding Metabolism

2.1. What is Metabolism and How it Works?

In the journey to uncover intermittent fasting, understanding metabolism, a key player that plays a fundamental role in our health and well-being, is crucial. Metabolism isn't just an isolated process; it's the sum of all the chemical reactions occurring in our body to keep the cells and organs alive.

Definition and Functions of Metabolism

Metabolism can be divided into two main categories: catabolism and anabolism. Catabolism is the process of breaking down molecules to produce energy. This includes the digestion of food and the conversion of nutrients into energy. Conversely, anabolism refers to the building of cellular components, such as proteins and nucleic acids, a process that requires energy.

These two processes are interdependent and balance each other to maintain the body in a state of homeostasis, or balance. Metabolism regulates vital functions such as body temperature, heart rate, the building and repair of tissues and organs, and the response to environmental stimuli.

Metabolism in the Context of Intermittent Fasting

In the context of intermittent fasting, metabolism takes on a central role. When the body enters a fasting state, a shift in metabolism occurs. After the glucose reserves in the blood and glycogen stored in muscles and the liver are depleted, the body begins to use stored fat as its primary source of energy, a process known as ketosis.

During ketosis, the body breaks down fats into fatty acids and ketone bodies. These ketone bodies serve as an alternative energy source for the brain and other vital organs. This shift from burning carbohydrates to fats for energy can have beneficial effects on various health aspects, including improved weight management, reduced inflammation, and potentially better cardiovascular health.

Basal Metabolic Rate and Physical Activity

The basal metabolic rate (BMR) is the amount of energy, expressed in calories, that the body requires to perform its basic functions at rest. Everyone has a unique BMR, influenced by factors such as age, sex, body composition, and genetics. Intermittent fasting can affect BMR, often leading to a more efficient metabolism.

Physical activity is another significant factor affecting metabolism. Regular exercise can increase BMR, improve insulin sensitivity, and increase muscle mass, which in turn burns more calories at rest compared to fat tissue.

Conclusion and Transition to the Next Section

Understanding metabolism is fundamental to grasp how intermittent fasting impacts our body and health. In the next section, we will delve deeper into the impact of intermittent fasting on metabolism, examining how this practice can optimize our metabolic function and help us achieve health and wellness goals.

2.2 Impact of Intermittent Fasting on Metabolism

Having defined metabolism and its basic functions, it's important to examine the specific impact that intermittent fasting has on this vital process. Intermittent fasting not only alters the way our body processes and utilizes energy but can also lead to significant improvements in metabolic health.

Metabolic Changes During Fasting

When we begin fasting, our body transitions from a fed state to a fasting state, a change that triggers a series of metabolic adaptations. Initially, the body uses stored glucose in the form of glycogen, primarily in the liver and muscles, as the primary source of energy. These glycogen reserves last for about 12-36 hours, after which the body begins to search for other energy sources.

Transition to Ketosis

Once glycogen reserves are depleted, the body enters a state called ketosis. In this state, the body starts burning stored fats for energy. This process involves breaking down fats into fatty acids and glycerol, which can be further converted into ketone bodies in the liver. Ketone bodies provide an efficient energy source for the brain and other tissues.

Effects on Insulin Sensitivity

Intermittent fasting can improve insulin sensitivity. During periods of food intake, insulin levels naturally increase to help transport blood glucose into cells. By fasting, these insulin spikes are reduced, which can help prevent insulin resistance, a condition that often precedes type 2 diabetes.

Improvement in Lipid Metabolism

Intermittent fasting positively affects lipid metabolism. By reducing meal frequency, the body has more time to process and use fats as energy, thus improving the lipid profile in the blood. This can reduce the risk of developing heart diseases and improve overall cardiovascular health.

Self-Regulation and Cellular Repair

During fasting, the body also has the opportunity to self-regulate and repair cells. This includes processes such as autophagy, where cells clean up and recycle damaged or non-functional components, improving cellular health and reducing the risk of some diseases.

Conclusion and Transition to the Next Section

The effect of intermittent fasting on metabolism is profound and multifactorial. From ketosis to insulin sensitivity, the benefits can have a significant impact on health and overall well-being. In the next section, we will explore the difference between basal and active metabolism, to understand how these two forms of metabolism react and adapt to intermittent fasting.

2.3. Basal Metabolism vs. Active Metabolism

After examining how intermittent fasting affects metabolism as a whole, it's crucial to delve deeper into the understanding of basal metabolism and active metabolism. This distinction helps us better understand how our body uses energy and how intermittent fasting can optimize these functions.

**What is Basal Metabolism? **

Basal Metabolic Rate (BMR) represents the amount of energy, measured in calories, that our body needs to maintain vital functions at rest. This includes activities such as breathing, blood circulation, body temperature regulation, cellular growth and repair, and organ function. BMR varies from person to person depending on factors such as age, sex, body composition, and genetics.

The Influence of Intermittent Fasting on Basal Metabolism

Intermittent fasting can have a direct impact on BMR. During fasting periods, the body requires less immediate energy, as it is not actively digesting food. This can lead to metabolic adaptability, where the body learns to use energy more efficiently. This efficiency may result in a slightly reduced BMR, but more effective at burning stored fats for energy.

**What is Active Metabolism? **

Conversely, active metabolism refers to the energy burned during activities beyond resting, such as walking, exercising, and even eating and digesting food. The rate at which we burn calories during these activities is known as the Active Metabolic Rate (AMR). AMR varies greatly depending on an individual's physical activity level and body composition.

Effects of Intermittent Fasting on Active Metabolism

Intermittent fasting can positively affect AMR. During fasting periods, the body may increase its use of fats for energy, which can lead to an increase in active metabolism, especially when combined with exercise. Additionally, intermittent fasting can improve insulin sensitivity and metabolic function, making the body more efficient at using energy during physical activities.

Balance Between Basal and Active Metabolism

Understanding the balance between BMR and AMR is crucial for optimizing the effects of intermittent fasting. A balanced approach to fasting and exercise can help maintain a healthy active metabolism while benefiting from an efficient basal metabolism. This balance is essential for supporting long-term weight loss and improving overall health.

Conclusion and Transition to the Next Section

Knowing the difference between basal and active metabolism allows us to understand how intermittent fasting can be used to optimize our overall metabolism. In the next section, we will delve deeper into how intermittent fasting optimizes metabolism, exploring strategies to maximize the metabolic benefits of this practice.

2.4. How Intermittent Fasting Optimizes Metabolism

Having explored basal and active metabolism, it's crucial to understand how intermittent fasting can optimize these aspects of metabolism. This optimization not only contributes to weight loss but also to the improvement of overall health and the prevention of chronic diseases.

Energy Efficiency and Metabolic Adaptation

One of the key aspects of metabolic optimization through intermittent fasting is the increase in the body's energy efficiency. During fasting periods, the body learns to use energy resources more effectively. This results in better management of fat reserves and more efficient use of glucose when available. This adaptation can lead to a more efficient metabolism even during non-fasting periods.

Improvement in Insulin Sensitivity

Intermittent fasting improves insulin sensitivity, a key factor in metabolism regulation. With optimized insulin sensitivity, cells respond better to insulin and manage blood glucose more effectively, reducing the risk of type 2 diabetes and improving overall energy metabolism.

Increased Fat Metabolism

Intermittent fasting prompts the body to switch from relying on carbohydrates as the primary energy source to using fats. This process, known as nutritional ketosis, not only aids in weight loss but also improves cardiovascular health and reduces inflammation.

Reduction of Oxidative Stress and Inflammation

Intermittent fasting can reduce oxidative stress and inflammation, two factors that negatively impact metabolism and overall health. By reducing these inflammatory processes, intermittent fasting contributes to cellular health and the prevention of chronic diseases.

Effects on Longevity and Disease Prevention

Studies have shown that intermittent fasting can positively affect longevity and reduce the risk of several chronic diseases. This is due in part to its ability to optimize metabolism, improve insulin sensitivity, and reduce inflammation.

Conclusion and Transition to the Next Section

In conclusion, intermittent fasting offers a range of benefits that extend beyond mere weight loss, optimizing metabolism so that it functions more effectively and efficiently. In the next section, we will explore the link between metabolism and weight loss, delving into how these metabolic changes contribute to sustainable results in the context of weight loss and overall well-being.

2.5. Link Between Metabolism and Weight Loss

After exploring how intermittent fasting optimizes metabolism, it's crucial to understand its direct impact on weight loss. Metabolism plays a pivotal role in regulating body weight, and the modifications brought about by intermittent fasting can have significant effects in this context.

The Role of Metabolism in Weight Loss

Metabolism determines the rate at which the body burns calories to produce energy. An efficient metabolism burns calories more effectively, even at rest, which can contribute to weight loss. Intermittent fasting, by optimizing metabolism, can thus speed up this process, making it easier for the body to use fat reserves as an energy source.

Intermittent Fasting and Energy Balance

The key concept in weight loss is the energy balance: the difference between energy intake (through food) and energy expenditure (through metabolism and physical activity). Intermittent fasting helps regulate this balance by reducing calorie intake during fasting periods and increasing metabolic efficiency. This combination can lead to a caloric deficit, which is essential for weight loss.

Effects of Intermittent Fasting on Fat Metabolism

As discussed previously, intermittent fasting induces the body to enter a state of ketosis, where fats are converted into energy. This process not only aids in reducing fat deposits but also improves lipid metabolism, further contributing to weight loss and cardiovascular health.

Preventing the Yo-Yo Effect

One of the advantages of intermittent fasting is its ability to prevent the yo-yo effect, common in many restrictive diets. Since intermittent fasting leads to a change in how the body uses energy, rather than drastically limiting calorie intake, the results are often more sustainable in the long term.

Intermittent Fasting: Beyond Weight Loss

It's important to highlight that intermittent fasting is not just a tool for weight loss but an approach to improving overall health. Beyond reducing body fat, it brings benefits such as improved insulin sensitivity, reduced inflammation, and potential increases in longevity.

Conclusion and Transition to the Next Chapter

In conclusion, the link between metabolism and weight loss is evident and significant in the context of intermittent fasting. By understanding this link, we can use intermittent fasting as an effective tool for weight management and improving metabolic health. In the next chapter, we will shift our focus to exploring the various forms of intermittent fasting, offering readers a guide on how to choose and implement the method that best suits their individual needs.

Chapter 3: Various Forms of Intermittent Fasting

3.1. Overview of Different Types of Intermittent Fasting

Entering the third chapter of our journey in "Natural and Rejuvenating Rhythms," we dive into the diversity of intermittent fasting practices. This flexible method of managing food intake has evolved into various forms, each with its peculiarities and benefits. Understanding the available options is essential for choosing the fasting method that best suits one's needs and goals.

Common Types of Intermittent Fasting

Intermittent fasting can be categorized based on the duration of fasting and eating periods. Here are some of the most common forms:

**The 16/8 Method: ** This is one of the most popular methods, where you fast for 16 hours and eat within an 8-hour window. For example, one might choose to eat between 12:00 PM and 8:00 PM, then fast until noon the next day.

**The 5:2 Method: ** In this practice, you eat normally for five days of the week, while for two non-consecutive days, you limit calorie intake to about 500-600 calories per day.

**Alternate-Day Fasting: ** As the name suggests, this method involves a full or partial fast every other day, alternated with days of normal or slightly increased eating.

**The Eat-Stop-Eat Method: ** This practice involves one or two days of complete fasting each week, going without food for 24 consecutive hours, for example, from dinner to dinner.

**The Warrior Diet: ** In this approach, you consume a small number of raw fruits and vegetables during the day and have a single, large meal in the evening.

Customizing Intermittent Fasting

Choosing a fasting method depends on various factors, such as lifestyle, health and weight goals, and personal preferences. Some may find it easier to start with less restrictive methods like the 16/8, while others may prefer the structure of alternate day fasting. It's important to listen to your body and adapt the fasting practice according to your needs and reactions.

Benefits and Considerations

Each method of intermittent fasting has its unique benefits. For example, the 16/8 method is often praised for its ease of integration into daily life, while the 5:2 may be more suited to those who prefer to limit calorie intake on specific days. Regardless of the chosen method, key benefits of intermittent fasting such as weight loss, improved metabolism, and increased insulin sensitivity are generally observed across all forms.

Conclusion and Transition to the Next Section

In conclusion, intermittent fasting offers a variety of methods that can be customized to fit different lifestyles and goals. In the next section, we will focus on the 16/8 method, exploring in detail how it works, its specific benefits, and how it can be effectively integrated into daily routines.

3.2. 16/8: 16-hour Fasting

After exploring various forms of intermittent fasting, the 16/8 method deserves special attention for its popularity and accessibility. This method, also known as the "fast/eat" eating pattern, involves a daily fast of 16 hours followed by an 8-hour eating period.

Principles of the 16/8 Method

The 16/8 method is based on the idea of limiting the eating period each day, allowing the body to enter a fasting state for a significant period. During the 16 hours of fasting, the body has the chance to deplete its glycogen reserves and start burning fats, a process that can lead to weight loss and improved metabolic health.

Practical Implementation

To start with the 16/8 method, it's important to choose an eating window that fits your lifestyle. For example, if you finish dinner at 8:00 PM, your next meal should be at 12:00 PM the following day. During the fasting hours, drinking water, tea, and unsweetened coffee is allowed, but caloric foods or beverages should be avoided.

Health and Weight Loss Benefits

The 16/8 method has been linked to numerous health benefits, including:

- **Weight Loss: ** By reducing the eating window, many people naturally consume fewer calories, facilitating a caloric deficit that leads to weight loss.

- **Improved Metabolism: ** Prolonged fasting can improve insulin sensitivity and promote a more efficient use of body fat as an energy source.

- **Cognitive Benefits: ** Some studies suggest that intermittent fasting may improve cognitive function and reduce the risk of neurodegenerative disorders.

Considerations and Adaptability

The 16/8 method is flexible and can be adapted to suit various needs and lifestyles. It's important to listen to your body and make any necessary adjustments. For instance, some people may find it beneficial to start with a shorter fasting period and gradually increase it.

Conclusion and Transition to the Next Section

The 16/8 method is an excellent starting point for those new to intermittent fasting. It offers a balance between flexibility and structure, making it sustainable in the long term. In the next section, we will explore another popular method, the 5:2, which proposes a different approach to intermittent fasting, focusing on caloric restriction for two days a week.

3.3. 5:2: Fasting for 2 Days a Week

Moving from a daily fasting approach like the 16/8, we now explore the 5:2 method, another popular intermittent fasting regime focusing on caloric restriction for two days a week.

Fundamental Concepts of the 5:2 Method

The 5:2 method involves five days of normal eating and two days of significant caloric restriction each week. During the restriction days, calorie intake is reduced to about 500-600 calories for women and 600-700 calories for men. These restriction days should not be consecutive to avoid excessive fatigue and stress on the body.

Implementation and Flexibility

The choice of fasting days in the 5:2 method is flexible and can be adapted based on lifestyle and personal commitments. It's crucial that on the calorie-restricted days, the food intake is nutritious, focusing on foods high in protein, fiber, and essential nutrients to maximize satiety and nutritional value.

Benefits of the 5:2 Method

The 5:2 method offers several health benefits, including:

- **Weight Loss: ** The weekly caloric restriction can lead to an overall caloric deficit, facilitating weight loss.

- **Improved Insulin Resistance: ** Similar to other fasting methods, the 5:2 can improve insulin sensitivity, reducing the risk of type 2 diabetes.

- **Mental Health Benefits: ** Some find that this method helps improve concentration and mental clarity during calorie-restricted days.

Nutritional Considerations

On fasting days of the 5:2 method, focusing on low glycemic index foods, high in fiber and protein, is essential. Vegetables, fruits, legumes, and lean proteins are excellent choices to ensure the body receives necessary nutrients while maintaining a low-calorie intake.

Conclusion and Transition to the Next Section

The 5:2 method offers a unique approach to intermittent fasting, allowing for greater flexibility and potentially greater sustainability long-term for some individuals. In the next section, we will examine alternate-day fasting, another form of intermittent fasting that proposes a different approach, alternating days of normal eating with days of complete or partial fasting.

3.4. Alternate-Day Fasting

After examining the 5:2 method, we move on to another intermittent fasting strategy: alternate day fasting. This approach proposes a fasting pattern that alternates days of normal eating with days of complete or partial fasting.

Principles of Alternate-Day Fasting

Alternate day fasting involves alternating between days where you eat normally and days where you consume few calories (around 500-600 for women and 600-700 for men) or no calories at all. This method is considered one of the more intense forms of intermittent fasting, but it can also offer significant results in terms of weight loss and health improvements.

Implementation and Flexibility

Alternate day fasting requires a degree of planning to ensure that fasting and eating days fit an individual's lifestyle. It's important to choose fasting days that don't coincide with social events or commitments that could make fasting more challenging. Here again, flexibility is key: some may prefer to fast completely on fasting days, while others may opt for light caloric restriction.

Health Benefits

Alternate-day fasting has been linked to numerous health benefits, including:

- **Effective Weight Loss: ** This method can lead to a significant weekly caloric deficit, contributing to effective weight loss.

- **Improved Insulin Sensitivity: ** Like other fasting regimes, it can improve insulin sensitivity and aid in managing type 2 diabetes.

- **Cardioprotective Effects: ** Some studies have indicated a potential improvement in cardiovascular health among those who practice alternate-day fasting.

Considerations for Sustainability

While alternate day fasting can be effective, it can also be challenging to maintain long-term. It's crucial to listen to your body and adapt the regime if necessary to ensure it remains sustainable and beneficial. Consulting with a physician or dietitian can be helpful, especially for those with pre-existing medical conditions.

Conclusion and Transition to the Next Section

Alternate day fasting offers a rigorous but potentially very effective approach to intermittent fasting. Like any method, it has its advantages and challenges, and its effectiveness depends on individual needs and preferences. Next, we will explore the Warrior Diet, another style of intermittent fasting that incorporates an even shorter eating period and a longer fasting window.

3.5. The Warrior Method

The Warrior Method represents another intriguing aspect of intermittent fasting. This approach combines an extended fasting period with a reduced eating window, primarily focused on the end of the day.

Foundations of the Warrior Method

The Warrior Method is characterized by a fasting window of about 20 hours followed by a 4-hour eating period. During the fasting hours, the consumption of small amounts of low-calorie foods, such as raw fruits and vegetables, is encouraged, followed by a substantial and nutritious meal during the eating period.

Practical Implementation

In the Warrior Method, it's crucial that the main meal is well-balanced and nutrient-dense to ensure that the body receives everything it needs in terms of vitamins, minerals, proteins, healthy fats, and carbohydrates. Since the eating window is brief, every food choice becomes significant to maximize nutritional intake.

Benefits and Considerations

This method is known for its benefits in terms of weight loss, improved concentration, and potential increase in longevity. However, it can be challenging, especially for those accustomed to eating frequently throughout the day. The key to success with the

Warrior Method is gradual introduction of the routine and careful listening to one's body.

Adaptation to Daily Life

The biggest challenge of the Warrior Method is adapting it to daily social and work life. It's important to plan so that the eating period fits social and work commitments, minimizing the impact on daily activities and maintaining a healthy balance.

Transition to the Next Chapter

In conclusion, the Warrior Method, with its emphasis on a long fasting period followed by a short eating period, offers a unique and intense approach to intermittent fasting. As we explore these different methodologies, it's clear that intermittent fasting can be highly customizable to fit various lifestyles and goals. In the next chapter, we will move from an overview of fasting methods to the important topic of preparation and planning for fasting, an essential step for anyone wanting to embark on this journey towards improved health.

Chapter 4: Planning and Preparing for Fasting

4.1. Preparing the Body and Mind for Fasting

As we approach the practical aspect of intermittent fasting, it's crucial to prepare both the body and mind for this transition. A holistic approach that considers both physical and psychological aspects is essential for a successful and sustainable fasting experience.

Physical Preparation

Gradual Adaptation

Starting with gradual changes is key to preparing the body for fasting. If the current habit includes various snacks or frequent meals, begin by reducing these snacks and gradually extending the hours between meals. This process helps the body to adapt to a longer interval of time without food, reducing potential discomforts like irritability or headaches.

Balanced Nutrition

Before starting a fasting regime, it's important to ensure that your diet is well-balanced. Optimal nutritional intake prepares the body by providing all the necessary vitamins, minerals, and other nutrients. A diet rich in vegetables, fruits, high-quality proteins, healthy fats, and complex carbohydrates is recommended.

Portion Control

For those aiming at intermittent fasting for weight loss, it's helpful to start being more aware of food portions during the eating windows. This helps to avoid overeating during non-fasting periods.

Mental Preparation

Setting Clear Goals

Understanding clearly why you choose to undertake intermittent fasting is crucial. Establishing realistic goals and clear motivations helps to maintain focus and discipline, especially during challenging moments.

Growth Mindset

Adopting a growth mindset and viewing fasting as a journey of personal discovery can be extremely beneficial. Embrace fasting as an opportunity to learn more about yourself, your eating habits, and your relationship with food.

Managing Expectations

It's important to have realistic expectations. The benefits of intermittent fasting are not immediate and take time. Being patient and kind to oneself during this adaptation process is crucial.

Conclusion and Transition to the Next Section

Adequately preparing both the body and mind is an essential step before starting any form of intermittent fasting. This preparation will ensure not only a more comfortable start but also greater long-term success. In the next section, we will explore how to create a personalized fasting plan, a fundamental step for integrating fasting into your daily routine effectively.

4.2. Creating a Personalized Fasting Plan

After preparing the body and mind, the next step in the intermittent fasting journey is creating a personalized fasting plan. This plan should be tailored to fit your lifestyle, needs, and goals, ensuring maximum effectiveness and sustainability.

Assessing Your Lifestyle

Starting by assessing your lifestyle is crucial. Consider your daily commitments, work routine, social and family life. For example, if evenings are typically busy, it might be more convenient to plan your eating window during the day. Similarly, if mornings are hectic, starting the day with fasting might be more manageable.

Choosing the Right Fasting Method

Based on your lifestyle assessment, choose the fasting method that best suits you. It could be 16/8, 5:2, alternate day fasting, or another method. It's important that the chosen method does not feel overly burdensome or in conflict with your daily life habits.

Planning and Consistency

Once you've selected the method, create a schedule. If you opt for 16/8, decide on the specific times for fasting and eating, and try to stick to these times as closely as possible. Consistency helps the body regulate itself and makes the process simpler from a psychological standpoint.

Listening to Your Body

While following your fasting plan, it's critical to listen to your body. Note how you feel during both fasting and eating periods. If you encounter issues such as excessive tiredness or irritability, it may be necessary to revise your plan.

Integration with Nutrition

Incorporate a nutritional strategy into your plan. During eating periods, ensure your meals are balanced and rich in essential nutrients. This not only supports your overall health but also helps maintain satiety during fasting periods.

Monitoring and Adjustment

Keep track of your progress and how you feel. This monitoring can include weight, body measurements, energy levels, and any other health indicator you find important. Be ready to adjust your plan based on the outcomes and your experiences.

Conclusion and Transition to the Next Section

Creating a personalized fasting plan is a critical step toward success in intermittent fasting. With a well-thought-out plan, you can maximize the benefits of fasting while maintaining your lifestyle and health. In the next section, we will explore dietary considerations during intermittent fasting, a crucial aspect to ensure your body receives the nourishment it needs.

4.3. Dietary Considerations During Intermittent Fasting

While adopting an intermittent fasting regimen, it's crucial to pay attention to the quality of your diet during eating windows. This approach ensures that the body receives all the necessary nutrients to function optimally, supporting both the fasting process and overall health and wellness goals.

Nutritional Priorities

Essential Nutrients

During eating periods, it's vital to focus on nutrient-rich foods. This includes a variety of fruits and vegetables, high-quality proteins, healthy fats, and complex carbohydrates. These foods provide vitamins, minerals, fiber, and other essential nutrients necessary to keep the body healthy and energized.

Balancing Macronutrients

A balanced diet in terms of proteins, fats, and carbohydrates is essential. Proteins are crucial for repair and muscle building, fats provide energy and support cellular health, and complex carbohydrates offer a sustainable energy source and help maintain satiety.

Hydration

Maintaining proper hydration is critical, especially during fasting periods. Water aids in body temperature regulation, nutrient transport, and waste removal. Drinking sufficient water can also help manage hunger and maintain good energy levels.

Calorie Management

Although intermittent fasting doesn't require strict calorie counting, being mindful of overall calorie intake is helpful. Consuming too little can lead to nutritional deficiencies and reduced energy, while eating too much can counteract weight loss goals.

Food Quality

Prioritizing food quality is as important as quantity. Whole, unprocessed foods should make up the majority of the diet. Avoid highly processed foods, added sugars, and unhealthy fats, which can negatively impact both general health and progress in intermittent fasting.

Adapting to Individual Needs

It's essential to tailor the diet to individual needs. This might mean increasing protein intake for those who are very active physically or including more complex carbohydrates for those requiring more energy throughout the day.

Conclusion and Transition to the Next Section

By considering these dietary guidelines, it's possible to optimize the benefits of intermittent fasting, ensuring that the body is nourished, satisfied, and capable of supporting both fasting periods and daily life. In the next section, we will explore useful tools and resources that can assist in the intermittent fasting journey, providing practical and motivational support.

4.4. Useful Tools and Resources

In the journey of intermittent fasting, utilizing the right tools and resources can make a significant difference. These aids can not only facilitate the process but also provide support, motivation, and useful insights to optimize the fasting experience.

Tracking Apps

Fasting Apps

There are several apps specifically designed for intermittent fasting that can help track your fasting and eating schedules. These apps often include timers, reminders, and calendars to help you stay on track with your fasting program.

Food Tracking Apps

Food tracking apps can be useful for recording nutritional and caloric intake. Even though intermittent fasting doesn't require strict calorie counting, keeping track of what you eat can be helpful to ensure nutritional balance and maintain awareness of eating habits.

Diaries and Journaling

Keeping a diary can be an effective way to record not just your meals and fasting times but also to note how you feel physically and mentally. This can help identify patterns, progress, and areas needing adjustments.

Educational Books and Guides

Intermittent Fasting Literature

Reading books and guides on intermittent fasting can provide a deeper understanding of the science and practice behind this methodology. This type of reading can also offer practical strategies and advice to overcome common challenges.

Cookbooks

Cookbooks focusing on nutritious and balanced meals can be particularly useful. These can assist in preparing meals that are both satisfying and in line with intermittent fasting goals.

Online Community and Support

Participating in online forums, support groups, or social media dedicated to intermittent fasting can provide a sense of community and accountability. Sharing experiences, challenges, and successes with others can be a source of motivation and learning.

Progress Measurement Tools

Scales and Body Composition Meters

Tools like smart scales or body composition meters can provide useful data on progress in terms of weight loss, body fat percentage, and other health indicators.

Health Monitoring Tools

Devices such as smartwatches or fitness bracelets can help monitor physical activity, sleep, and other health parameters that can be influenced by intermittent fasting.

Conclusion and Transition to the Next Section

Utilizing these tools and resources can significantly increase the chances of success in intermittent fasting, providing support, guidance, and monitoring. In the next section, we will discuss managing expectations and setting goals in the context of intermittent fasting, an essential aspect of maintaining a balanced and realistic perspective on your journey towards wellness.

4.5. Managing Expectations and Setting Goals

A fundamental part of an effective approach to intermittent fasting is the proper management of expectations and setting realistic goals. This approach helps to maintain motivation and ensure that the fasting journey is sustainable and rewarding.

Understanding the Realistic Timing of Results

Avoid Expecting Immediate Results

While intermittent fasting can lead to significant outcomes, it's important not to expect drastic immediate changes. Weight loss and other health benefits occur gradually. Expecting instant improvements can lead to disappointment and frustration.

Recognizing Fluctuations

During the intermittent fasting journey, there will be ups and downs. Understanding that body weight and physical performance can fluctuate day-to-day helps maintain a balanced perspective.

Setting Specific and Measurable Goals

Short and Long-term Goals

Setting both short and long-term goals can provide clear benchmarks and maintain motivation. Short-term goals can be weekly or monthly, while long-term goals may look ahead several months or a year.

Goals Beyond Weight Loss

While weight loss may be a common goal, it's important to consider other benefits such as improvements in sleep, energy, concentration, and overall health.

Tailoring Goals to Your Needs

Customization

Adapt your goals to your personal circumstances, including health conditions, lifestyle, and limitations. Goals need to be realistic and achievable to be effective.

Evaluation and Adjustment

Periodically evaluate your progress and be ready to adjust your goals if necessary. This can include adapting the fasting method, adjusting eating windows, or changing dietary habits.

Encouraging a Positive Mindset

Celebrating Small Successes

Recognizing and celebrating small milestones along the way helps build confidence and motivation. Every step forward, no matter how small, is progress towards your overall goal.

Avoiding Comparison

Avoid comparing your progress with others. Each person is unique, and so will be their paths and results in intermittent fasting.

Conclusion and Transition to the Next Chapter

Managing expectations and setting realistic goals is essential for a successful journey in intermittent fasting. This approach ensures that you stay focused and motivated, celebrating the progress made. In the next chapter, we will delve into how intermittent fasting facilitates weight loss, exploring strategies to maximize this aspect.

Chapter 5: Losing Weight with Intermittent Fasting

5.1. How Intermittent Fasting Facilitates Weight Loss

Weight loss is one of the most common goals for those adopting intermittent fasting. Understanding how this practice facilitates weight loss is essential for using it effectively.

Weight Loss Mechanisms in Intermittent Fasting

Regulation of Energy Balance

Intermittent fasting helps to create a caloric deficit, which is crucial for weight loss. By alternating periods of eating with periods of fasting, one often reduces overall caloric intake without having to count every calorie.

Improvement in Insulin Sensitivity

During fasting, insulin levels decrease. This reduction improves insulin sensitivity, facilitating the body's process of using the glucose in the blood. Better insulin sensitivity helps to prevent fat accumulation and promotes a more efficient use of energy.

Increase in Fat Metabolism

Intermittent fasting encourages the body to use fat reserves for energy, a process known as lipolysis. This is particularly evident during ketosis, a metabolic state achieved during prolonged periods of fasting.

Effects on Growth Hormone

Fasting can increase levels of growth hormone, which has beneficial effects on body composition. Growth hormone helps build lean muscle mass and burn fats, both essential for effective weight loss.

Practical Strategies for Maximizing Weight Loss

Selecting the Fasting Method

Choosing the fasting method that best suits your lifestyle and goals can significantly affect weight loss effectiveness. For instance, some people may find the 16/8 method more manageable and thus more effective long-term.

Focus on Food Quality

During eating windows, it's important to focus on the quality of foods. A nutrient-rich diet, with a good balance of proteins, healthy fats, and complex carbohydrates, can support the weight loss process.

Integrating Physical Activity

Physical activity, especially aerobic exercise and resistance training can further increase the caloric deficit and improve body composition. Regular exercise should be a key component of your weight loss plan.

Important Considerations

Listening to Your Body

It's crucial to listen to your body and adjust the fasting plan if necessary. If symptoms such as excessive tiredness or irritability are experienced, it may be necessary to review the fasting method or dietary strategy.

Long-term Sustainability

The key to successful weight loss is sustainability. Choosing an intermittent fasting approach that fits your lifestyle and personal preferences increases the likelihood of adhering to the plan long-term.

Conclusion and Transition to the Next Section

Intermittent fasting offers an effective means to facilitate weight loss through various physiological mechanisms and behavioral changes. By understanding these principles, one can maximize weight loss effectiveness. In the next section, we will explore specific strategies to maximize weight loss in the context of intermittent fasting.

5.2. Strategies to Maximize Weight Loss

Once the basic mechanisms through which intermittent fasting facilitates weight loss are understood, it's important to explore specific strategies to maximize this process. These strategies can help optimize results and maintain weight loss over time.

Careful Meal Planning

Nutritional Balance

During eating windows, focus on well-balanced meals that include a variety of essential nutrients. Each meal should contain a good source of lean protein, healthy fats, and complex carbohydrates. This approach supports not only weight loss but also overall health.

Preventing Overeating

Avoiding overeating during eating windows is crucial. Even during non-fasting periods, it's important to listen to the body's hunger and fullness signals and avoid eating more than necessary.

Regular Physical Exercise

Combining Cardio and Strength Training

An exercise program that combines both cardiovascular activity and strength training can significantly increase fat loss. While cardio helps burn calories, strength training builds muscle which enhances basal metabolism.

Exercise Timing

Experiment with the timing of physical activity. Some find it beneficial to exercise during the eating window, while others prefer working out during fasting periods to enhance lipolysis.

Stress and Sleep Management

Stress Control

High stress levels can negatively impact weight loss by increasing appetite and promoting fat deposition, especially in the abdominal area. Stress management techniques such as meditation, yoga, or deep breathing can be beneficial.

Importance of Sleep

Adequate sleep is vital for effective weight loss. Lack of sleep can disrupt the hormones that regulate hunger and increase cravings for high-calorie foods.

Hydration

Calorie-Free Beverages

Drinking plenty of water and maintaining proper hydration is crucial. Water can help manage hunger and boost metabolism. During fasting periods, calorie-free beverages like water, tea, and unsweetened coffee are recommended.

Listening to Your Body

Individual Adaptations

Recognize that everybody reacts differently. If a strategy isn't working for you, don't hesitate to modify it. Listening to your body is key to finding what works best.

Conclusion and Transition to the Next Section

By adopting these strategies, you can maximize weight loss through intermittent fasting. In the next section, we will examine how to avoid common weight loss pitfalls, an important aspect of maintaining long-term benefits.

5.3. Avoiding Common Weight Loss Pitfalls

In the journey towards weight loss with intermittent fasting, it's easy to fall into some common traps. Being aware of these obstacles can help avoid them and maintain steady and healthy progress.

Unrealistic Expectations

Avoiding the "All-or-Nothing" Mentality

One of the most common mistakes is having unrealistic expectations, such as losing weight too quickly. This can lead to frustration and an extreme "all-or-nothing" approach that often ends with abandoning the fasting plan.

Setting Realistic Goals

Setting realistic and achievable weight loss goals is crucial. Remember, sustainable weight loss happens gradually. A weight reduction of about 0.5-1 kg per week is generally considered healthy and sustainable.

Underestimating Caloric Intake

Watch Out for "Free" Meals

During eating windows, it can be easy to underestimate caloric intake. Even though intermittent fasting doesn't rely on calorie counting, it's important to be aware of the quantity and quality of food consumed.

Nutritional Balance

Ensure your meals are well-balanced. Consuming too many high-calorie density foods without sufficient nutrients can hinder weight loss.

Neglecting Other Health Aspects

Importance of Physical Exercise

Weight loss isn't just about diet. Regular physical exercise is an essential component for effective weight loss and for improving overall health.

Mental and Emotional Health

Mental and emotional health play a significant role in weight loss. Stress and sleep disorders can negatively impact metabolism and eating habits.

Lack of Support

Seeking Support

The weight loss journey can be challenging to tackle alone. Having a support system, whether it be a fasting group, friends, family, or a professional, can provide encouragement and accountability.

Using Online Communities

Online communities can offer advice, support, and the sharing of experiences with others on similar paths.

Relaxing Too Much in Later Stages

Maintaining Consistency

Even after achieving significant weight loss results, it's important to maintain consistency in the fasting regime and healthy eating habits.

Avoiding Complacency

Don't let yourself become complacent. Continue to monitor your progress and stay true to the practices that have led to success.

Conclusion and Transition to the Next Section

By avoiding these common pitfalls, you can maximize your weight loss and maintain the results over time. In the next section, we will explore success stories and testimonials, which can provide further motivation and inspiration on your weight loss journey with intermittent fasting.

5.4. Success Stories and Testimonials

Success stories and testimonials are powerful sources of inspiration and motivation, especially in the context of intermittent fasting. Hearing or reading about others' positive experiences can affirm that intermittent fasting can be an effective path to better health and weight loss.

Variety in Experiences

Success stories in intermittent fasting are as diverse as the people who tell them. These stories can range from significant weight loss to improvements in overall health, increased energy, and mental well-being. This variety demonstrates the adaptability of intermittent fasting to different needs and lifestyles.

Common Elements in Success Stories

Consistency and Patience

Many success stories emphasize the importance of consistency and patience. Individuals often recount how they had to gradually adapt to intermittent fasting and how, over time, they began to see positive changes.

Overcoming Challenges

The theme of overcoming challenges, such as managing hunger, adjusting to changes in eating routines, and resisting temptations, is also common. Hearing how others have faced and conquered these challenges can be extremely motivating.

Sustainable Lifestyle

Another recurring theme in success stories is the sustainability of intermittent fasting as a lifestyle, rather than a temporary diet. Many people describe how intermittent fasting has become a natural part of their daily routine.

Psychological Impact

Increased Self-Confidence

Hearing how others have improved their self-esteem and confidence through intermittent fasting can be particularly inspiring. These changes can result not only from weight loss but also from improved overall health and a sense of control over one's well-being.

Changes in Relationship with Food

Testimonials often highlight how intermittent fasting has changed one's relationship with food, leading to heightened awareness and more mindful choices.

Sharing and Community

Participating in online communities or support groups where people share their stories can provide a sense of belonging and understanding. Listening to or sharing experiences can reinforce determination and offer new ideas or strategies for addressing personal challenges.

Conclusion and Transition to the Next Section

Success stories and testimonials offer not just proof of the effectiveness of intermittent fasting but also valuable lessons and inspiration. In the next section, we will examine how to sustain long-term weight loss, a crucial aspect of maintaining the benefits achieved through intermittent fasting.

5.5. Sustaining Long-term Weight Loss

Maintaining long-term weight loss is perhaps the most significant challenge in the intermittent fasting journey. It's crucial to adopt strategies that not only facilitate initial weight loss but also help sustain these results over time.

Adopting Intermittent Fasting as a Lifestyle

Beyond Dieting

Long-term success with intermittent fasting requires seeing it not as a temporary diet but as a lifestyle change. This involves integrating fasting into your daily routine sustainably and comfortably.

Flexibility and Adaptability

Flexibility is key. Being willing to adapt your fasting plan based on changes in your lifestyle, health, and goals is important for long-term sustainability.

Continuous Monitoring and Evaluation

Regular Review of Goals

Periodically assessing your progress and goals is essential. This can include tracking weight but also other health indicators such as energy levels, sleep quality, and overall well-being.

Adjustments Based on Results

Be ready to make adjustments to your fasting plan or dietary strategy based on the results you're achieving and how you're feeling.

Maintaining Nutritional Balance

Importance of a Balanced Diet

Continue to focus on a balanced diet during eating windows. Consuming a variety of nutrient-rich foods is crucial for keeping the body healthy and preventing nutritional deficiencies.

Avoiding Excessive Restrictions

Avoid imposing overly strict dietary restrictions. A too restrictive diet can be hard to maintain long-term and can lead to nutritional deficiencies and an unhealthy relationship with food.

Stress and Sleep Management

Stress Reduction Techniques

Implement regular practices to manage stress, such as meditation, breathing exercises, or recreational activities. Excessive stress can compromise weight loss and overall well-being.

Prioritizing Quality Sleep

Ensure you're getting sufficient quality sleep. Lack of sleep can negatively impact hunger hormones and make it more difficult to maintain weight loss.

Building Sustainable Support

Support Network

Maintaining or building a support network, including friends, family, or online groups, can provide encouragement and useful advice.

Sharing and Learning

Sharing experiences and learning from others can offer new perspectives and strategies for addressing common challenges in maintaining weight loss.

Conclusion and Transition to the Next Chapter

Through these approaches, the weight loss achieved with intermittent fasting can be effectively maintained in the long term. In the next chapter, we will focus on identifying and overcoming common challenges in intermittent fasting, a crucial aspect of sustaining progress over time.

Chapter 6: Overcoming the Challenges of Intermittent Fasting

6.1. Identifying and Managing Common Obstacles

Success in intermittent fasting involves not only good planning and strategy but also the ability to recognize and overcome common obstacles that may arise along the way. This section explores typical challenges and provides tips on how to tackle them.

Adjustment Phase

Dealing with Initial Discomfort

In the beginning stages of intermittent fasting, it's common to experience discomfort such as hunger, headaches, or irritability. It's important to recognize that these are often signs of the body's adjustment phase. To manage them, start gradually, slowly increasing the fasting duration.

Listening to Your Body

Listening attentively to your body during this period is crucial. If symptoms are too intense, it may be necessary to revise your fasting plan or consult a healthcare professional.

Dietary Challenges

Managing Cravings

Cravings for specific foods can be a challenge, especially during the fasting period. To tackle them, ensure your meals are nutritious and filling, and try to determine if cravings are driven by habits or emotions.

Avoiding Overeating

Avoiding overeating during eating windows is crucial. Focus on the quality of food rather than quantity, and practice listening actively to your body's hunger and fullness signals.

Emotional and Mental Obstacles

Overcoming Mental Barriers

Mental challenges such as lack of motivation or feeling discouraged can arise, especially in the face of slow or stagnant progress. To overcome them, remember why you started intermittent fasting and celebrate small successes along the way.

Managing Stress and Anxiety

Stress and anxiety can interfere with intermittent fasting, often leading to emotional eating. Find healthy ways to manage stress, such as exercise, meditation, or engaging in relaxing hobbies.

Social Impacts

Navigating Social Situations

Social situations, like dinners or events, can pose a challenge, especially when they coincide with the fasting period. Plan ahead, choosing to adjust your eating window or consciously deciding to make an exception for that event.

Support from Friends and Family

Communicating with friends and family about your goals and fasting schedule can help gain their support and understanding.

Conclusion and Transition to the Next Section

Recognizing and managing these challenges is a crucial step in maintaining long-term success in intermittent fasting. In the next section, we will specifically explore how to handle hunger and food cravings during fasting, one of the most common challenges faced on this journey.

6.2. Tips for Managing Hunger and Food Cravings

Managing hunger and cravings is one of the most common challenges in intermittent fasting. Effectively addressing these moments can make a difference in maintaining a sustainable and rewarding fasting journey.

Understanding Hunger

Physical Hunger vs. Emotional Hunger

Distinguishing between physical hunger and emotional hunger is crucial. While physical hunger is a natural need of the body, emotional hunger is often triggered by stress, boredom, or habits. Recognizing the type of hunger can help make more mindful food choices.

Listening to Body Signals

Learn to recognize your body's signals. Physical hunger develops gradually and is satisfied with eating, whereas emotional hunger appears suddenly and craves specific, often unhealthy, foods.

Strategies for Managing Hunger

Hydration

Drinking plenty of water can help manage hunger, as the body sometimes confuses thirst with hunger. Drinking a glass of water when you feel hungry can provide a pause to assess whether the hunger is real or emotional.

Foods Rich in Fiber and Proteins

Include foods rich in fiber and proteins during your eating windows. These nutrients help maintain satiety longer, reducing hunger during fasting periods.

Distraction and Activities

Finding ways to distract yourself or engage in an activity can be a great way to get through moments of intense hunger. Physical activity, reading, or a hobby can divert attention away from food.

Managing Cravings

Identifying Triggers

Understanding what triggers your cravings is the first step to managing them. This can include emotional, environmental factors, or certain habitual patterns.

Healthy Alternatives

Having healthy snacks available can help satisfy cravings without compromising your fasting goals. These snacks should be nutritious and low in calories, such as fruits, vegetables, nuts, or Greek yogurt.

Mindfulness Techniques

Practicing mindfulness can help manage cravings. This can include deep breathing techniques, meditation, or simply taking a moment to reflect on the reasons behind your craving.

Conclusion and Transition to the Next Section

Effectively managing hunger and cravings is a crucial element for success in intermittent fasting. By implementing these strategies, you can navigate these challenging moments and keep your fasting journey on track. In the next section, we will examine how to maintain motivation and self-control, two fundamental aspects of persevering in intermittent fasting.

6.3. Maintaining Motivation and Self-Control

Maintaining motivation and self-control is crucial in pursuing any long-term goal, particularly true in the case of intermittent fasting. These aspects can often be the key to overcoming challenges and staying on track.

Identifying Intrinsic Motivation

Discovering the "Why"

Understanding your personal and deep reason for choosing intermittent fasting can serve as a powerful motivator. Whether it's improving health, losing weight, or increasing energy, having a clear "why" helps stay focused even in tough times.

Setting Personal Goals

Set goals that are meaningful to you. Goals should be Specific, Measurable, Achievable, Relevant, and Time-bound (SMART) to maximize the likelihood of success.

Creating a Sustainable Routine

Integration into Lifestyle

Adapting the fasting regimen to fit your lifestyle, rather than the other way around, increases the chances of long-term adherence. A routine that fits well into your daily life is less likely to require excessive self-control.

Regularity and Predictability

Maintaining a degree of regularity and predictability in your fasting routine can help reduce the stress and decision fatigue associated with choosing when and what to eat.

Using Self-Control Techniques

Advance Planning

Planning meals and fasting windows in advance can help avoid impulsive decisions that could hinder your progress.

Distraction Techniques

When cravings or temptation arise, use distraction techniques such as taking a walk, reading a book, or engaging in a hobby to shift focus.

External Support and Accountability

Support Network

Building a support network of friends, family, or other individuals on a similar path can offer encouragement and accountability.

Online Groups and Communities

Joining groups or online communities dedicated to intermittent fasting can provide a constant source of motivation and useful advice.

Reflection and Self-Evaluation

Tracking Progress

Keeping track of progress, both physical and emotional, can be a powerful motivator. This can include tracking weight, body measurements, or simply noting how you feel.

Adaptation and Flexibility

Being willing to adjust your approach based on results and personal experiences is important. Flexibility can prevent frustration and keep the process more manageable.

Conclusion and Transition to the Next Section

Maintaining motivation and self-control in intermittent fasting requires a mix of personal strategies, external support, and a good dose of self-awareness. In the next section, we will discuss social and community support in intermittent fasting, another critical aspect of a successful and lasting practice.

6.4. Social and Community Support in Fasting

Social and community support plays a crucial role in maintaining motivation and adherence to intermittent fasting. Having a support network can make the journey less isolating and more rewarding.

Importance of Social Support

Sense of Belonging

Feeling part of a community that shares the same goals can be immensely reassuring. Knowing you're not alone in your daily challenges can boost motivation and willpower.

Exchange of Advice and Strategies

Interacting with others allows for the exchange of advice, tips, and strategies that have worked for others. This type of collective learning is invaluable, especially for those new to intermittent fasting.

Finding or Creating Support Groups

Online Groups and Forums

Forums and online groups, such as those on social platforms like Facebook, Reddit, or specialized forums, offer a place to share experiences, ask questions, and receive support.

Local Groups and Meetups

Participating in local groups or meetups can provide more personalized support. Meeting people in person to share experiences can be particularly motivating.

Overcoming Social Challenges

Managing Social Situations

Navigating social situations, such as dinners or parties, can be challenging with intermittent fasting. Discussing your fasting regimen in advance with friends and family can help mitigate awkwardness and find compromises.

Involving Friends and Family

Explaining the benefits and workings of intermittent fasting to friends and family can lead to their understanding and, possibly, their active support in your journey.

Emotional Benefits of Support

Stress Reduction

Knowing you have a support network can significantly reduce the stress associated with changing eating habits and lifestyle.

Positive Reinforcement

Receiving positive reinforcement from group members can increase self-esteem and confidence in your ability to adhere to intermittent fasting.

Conclusion and Transition to the Next Section

Social and community support in intermittent fasting not only provides a source of encouragement and advice but can also be a powerful tool for overcoming challenges and achieving your goals. In the next section, we will explore when it might be necessary to pause or adjust fasting, a crucial consideration to ensure that the practice remains healthy and beneficial.

6.5. Recognizing When to Pause or Modify Fasting

In the journey of intermittent fasting, it's essential to recognize the signs indicating the need to pause or modify the fasting regimen. Attentively listening to your body and responding to its signals can prevent health issues and ensure that fasting remains a healthy and sustainable practice.

Physical Signals to Monitor

Feeling Excessively Tired or Weak

If you start to feel regularly tired or weak, it could be a sign that your body isn't adapting well to fasting. This can be particularly true if the fatigue disrupts daily activities or physical exercise.

Digestive Problems

Issues like chronic constipation, diarrhea, or abdominal discomfort can be signals that intermittent fasting is negatively impacting your digestion.

Mood Variations and Irritability

Changes in mood, such as irritability or depression, can be signs that fasting is negatively affecting your mental health.

Emotional and Mental Signals

Obsession with Food and Meals

If you find that fasting leads you to become obsessed with food or upcoming meals, it might be time to review your approach.

Feeling Overwhelmed or Stressed

If fasting adds significant stress to your life, it might not be the right time to engage in this practice.

General Health Considerations

Monitoring Pre-existing Conditions

If you have pre-existing health conditions, it's crucial to closely monitor their symptoms. In some cases, fasting may need adjustment to not exacerbate these conditions.

Consulting Healthcare Professionals

If you suspect that fasting is negatively affecting your health, it's important to consult a doctor or a dietitian. They can provide personalized advice and help you decide whether to continue, modify, or stop fasting.

Adapting the Fasting Regimen

Modifying the Duration of Fasting

If you find fasting too challenging, consider reducing the duration of fasting periods or changing the fasting method.

Listening to Your Body

Being open to making adjustments based on how you feel is vital. Intermittent fasting should enhance your health and well-being, not diminish it.

Conclusion and Transition to the Next Chapter

Attentively listening to your body and recognizing the signals indicating the need to pause or modify fasting is essential to maintaining this practice as beneficial and healthy. In the next chapter, we will explore how intermittent fasting fits into an overall wellness and health strategy, emphasizing the importance of a holistic approach.

Chapter 7: Long-Term Benefits of Intermittent Fasting

7.1. Integrating Fasting into a Holistic Approach to Health and Wellness

Intermittent fasting, to be truly effective, should be integrated into a holistic approach to health and wellness. This means considering it not just as a weight loss method but as part of an overall strategy to improve the quality of life.

Beyond Weight Loss

Overall Physical Health

While intermittent fasting can aid in weight loss, its benefits can extend to many other aspects of physical health, such as improved insulin sensitivity, reduced inflammation, and enhanced cardiovascular health.

Disease Prevention and Management

Intermittent fasting can play a role in the prevention and management of certain chronic conditions, like type 2 diabetes, some forms of cancer, and heart diseases.

Mental and Emotional Health

Improving Mental Clarity

Many practitioners of intermittent fasting report improvements in mental clarity and concentration. This can be attributed to various factors, including reduced inflammation and a better energy balance.

Stress and Mood Management

Fasting can positively affect mood and stress management. However, it's important to monitor these aspects and ensure that fasting does not add additional stress to life.

Diet and Nutrition

Importance of a Balanced Diet

A nutritious and balanced diet is crucial. Intermittent fasting should be combined with healthy food choices to maximize health benefits and support long-term weight loss.

Listening to the Body

Listening to your body's signals regarding nutritional needs is essential. Adapting your diet to these needs helps maintain energy and overall well-being.

Physical Exercise and Activity

Regular Exercise

Integrating regular physical exercise into the intermittent fasting regime can amplify its benefits. Physical activity, both aerobic and strength, is important for heart health, weight management, and overall well-being.

Variety of Activities

Incorporating a variety of physical activities can keep exercise interesting and beneficial. This includes activities like walking, swimming, yoga, and weight training.

Holistic Wellness

Lifestyle Considerations

A holistic approach to wellness also includes other lifestyle aspects, such as adequate sleep, stress management, and maintaining healthy social relationships.

Listening to Your Body

Being in tune with the needs of your body and mind is crucial. This includes recognizing when it's necessary to rest, change habits, or seek professional support.

Conclusion and Transition to the Next Section

By integrating intermittent fasting into a holistic approach to health, you can not only lose weight but also improve the overall quality of life. In the next section, we will explore how intermittent fasting can be adapted to different life stages, ensuring it remains a healthy and flexible approach to changing needs.

7.2. Adapting Intermittent Fasting to Different Life Stages

Intermittent fasting can be a powerful tool for improving health and managing weight, but it's crucial to recognize that the body's needs can change at different life stages. Adapting fasting to these variations can ensure it remains a healthy and effective method.

Intermittent Fasting in Young Adults

Energy and Growth

For young adults, intermittent fasting needs to balance energy and growth requirements. Ensuring adequate nutrient intake to support an active lifestyle and physical development is important.

Building Healthy Habits

This life stage is an ideal opportunity to build healthy eating and exercise habits. Intermittent fasting can help develop body awareness and its nutritional needs.

Intermittent Fasting in Middle Age

Metabolism and Health

As age advances, metabolism tends to slow down. Intermittent fasting can be an effective way to manage weight and support metabolic health but should be accompanied by a nutritious diet and regular physical activity.

Disease Prevention

At this stage, preventing diseases like type 2 diabetes and heart diseases becomes a priority. Intermittent fasting can play a role in reducing risk factors for these conditions.

Intermittent Fasting During Pregnancy and Breastfeeding

Consulting a Healthcare Professional

During pregnancy and breastfeeding, the body's nutritional needs significantly increase. Consulting a doctor before starting or continuing an intermittent fasting regimen during these periods is essential.

Focus on Nutrition

If approved by a healthcare professional, intermittent fasting during these times should particularly emphasize adequate and balanced nutrition to support the health of both mother and child.

Adapting Fasting to Specific Health Conditions

Listening to the Body and Medical Advice

For those with specific health conditions, such as metabolic diseases or eating disorders, it's crucial to listen carefully to one's body and follow healthcare professionals' advice regarding intermittent fasting.

Personalized Adaptations

In some cases, specific adaptations may be necessary, such as reducing the fasting duration or modifying its frequency, to ensure the practice is safe and effective.

Conclusion and Transition to the Next Section

Adapting intermittent fasting to different life stages ensures that this practice remains beneficial and sustainable. In the next section, we will examine the importance of balancing intermittent fasting with adequate nutrition, a crucial aspect of maximizing the benefits of this practice.

7.3. Balancing Fasting with Adequate Nutrition

While intermittent fasting is an effective approach for health and weight loss, balancing it with adequate nutrition is crucial. This balance ensures the body receives all the necessary nutrients to function optimally while benefiting from fasting phases.

Importance of Nutritional Balance

Preventing Nutritional Deficiencies

During eating windows, focusing on the quality and variety of foods to prevent nutritional deficiencies is essential. A diet rich in fruits, vegetables, lean proteins, healthy fats, and complex carbohydrates provides a broad spectrum of essential nutrients.

Supporting Metabolism and Overall Health

A balanced diet supports metabolism, aids in weight regulation, and contributes to overall health, including immune function and mental health.

Meal Planning During Intermittent Fasting

Meal Planning Strategies

Planning meals in advance can help ensure you consume a variety of nutrient-rich foods. Consider including foods from all food groups and using spices and herbs to enhance flavor without adding excessive calories.

Portion Control

During eating windows, paying attention to portion sizes is important. Eating too much or too little can compromise both fasting goals and nutritional objectives.

Incorporating Dietary Variety

Dietary Diversity

Including a wide range of foods in your diet not only provides a range of essential nutrients but can also make eating more enjoyable and less monotonous.

Listening to Body Needs

Being attentive to your body's signals can help guide food choices. For example, if you feel tired, you may need more complex carbohydrates or iron in your diet.

Special Considerations

Adaptations for Physical Activity

If you are very physically active, you may need to increase your calorie intake or adjust the timing of your meals to ensure adequate energy and muscle recovery.

Adapting to Individual Needs

Recognize that nutritional needs can vary widely among different individuals. Factors such as age, gender, health status, activity level, and personal goals influence the type of nutrition needed.

Conclusion and Transition to the Next Section

A careful balance between fasting and adequate nutrition is key to maximizing the benefits of intermittent fasting. In the next section, we will explore how to integrate intermittent fasting with other wellness practices for a holistic approach to health.

7.4. Integrating Intermittent Fasting with Other Wellness Practices

To maximize the benefits of intermittent fasting, it's beneficial to integrate it with other wellness practices. This holistic approach can not only enhance the results of fasting but also contribute to a general sense of health and well-being.

Physical Exercise

Complementarity with Physical Activity

Physical activity is a natural complement to intermittent fasting. Regular exercise, both aerobic and strength training, can improve body composition, increase the efficacy of fasting, and promote overall health.

Exercise Timing

Experiment with the timing of exercise in relation to your fasting schedule. Some find exercising during their eating window to be more effective, while others prefer working out during fasting to enhance fat burning.

Stress Management and Sleep

Stress Reduction Techniques

Integrating stress-reduction practices such as meditation, yoga, or mindfulness can help manage stress, which in turn can positively influence the effectiveness of intermittent fasting.

Prioritizing Quality Sleep

Ensuring adequate sleep is crucial. Good nighttime rest supports physical and mental regeneration, directly affecting energy, metabolism, and the ability to sustain fasting.

Diet and Hydration

Balanced and Nutrient-Rich Diet

Incorporating a nutrient-rich and varied diet is essential. A diet that includes a wide variety of fruits, vegetables, lean proteins, healthy fats, and whole carbohydrates can provide the energy and nutrients needed to support fasting.

Adequate Hydration

Maintaining adequate hydration is crucial, especially during fasting periods. Drinking plenty of water, unsweetened tea, or infusions can help manage hunger and keep the body hydrated.

Integrating Holistic Health Practices

Holistic Approaches to Health

Exploring other holistic health practices such as acupuncture, reflexology, or nature-based therapies can offer additional benefits and help create a more comprehensive approach to wellness.

Enjoying Recreational Activities

Including recreational activities and hobbies that you enjoy can improve mental health and overall satisfaction, thus supporting your commitment to intermittent fasting.

Conclusion and Transition to the Next Section

Integrating intermittent fasting with various wellness practices creates a holistic approach to health. This combination can lead to better overall well-being and more lasting results. In the next section, we will explore the role of self-management and self-awareness in the success of intermittent fasting.

7.5. The Role of Self-Management and Self-Awareness in the Success of Intermittent Fasting

The success in intermittent fasting largely depends on an individual's ability to self-manage and have profound self-awareness. These skills allow customizing the fasting approach, proactively responding to changes, and maintaining a long-term commitment.

Developing Self-Awareness

Listening to Your Body

Learning to listen to your body's signals is crucial. This includes recognizing true hunger, understanding emotional responses to food, and identifying how different foods and fasting patterns affect well-being.

Personal Reflection

Regular reflection on your fasting experiences can help identify what aspects work well and what needs adjustment. Keeping a diary or a blog can be a useful tool for this reflection.

Effective Self-Management

Planning and Preparation

Effective planning and preparation are crucial. This might mean preparing meals in advance, planning fasting windows around social and work commitments, and setting reminders for the start and end times of fasting periods.

Proactive Challenge Management

Being proactive in managing challenges, such as cravings or changes in schedule, is essential. This requires a flexible mindset and the ability to adapt to changing circumstances.

Responding to Physical and Emotional Variations

Responding to Physical and Emotional Changes

Being aware of how your body and mind react over time to intermittent fasting is important. Recognizing changes in sleep, energy, mood, or stress levels may indicate the need to adjust your approach.

Adaptations Based on Age and Health Conditions

As life stages and health conditions change, your approach to fasting might need adaptations. For example, nutritional needs and metabolism change with age, requiring potential adjustments in the fasting regime.

Importance of External Support

Utilizing a Support Network

While self-management is key, leaning on a support network—whether friends, family, online groups, or health professionals—can provide guidance, advice, and encouragement.

Continuous Learning

Staying open to learning, both through personal resources and expert advice, is a key component of effective self-management in intermittent fasting.

Conclusion and Transition to the Next Section

Self-awareness and self-management are powerful tools in intermittent fasting, enabling a personalized and adaptable approach that responds to the changing needs of the body and mind. In the next chapter, we'll focus on specific dietary advice and recipe suggestions to maximize the benefits of intermittent fasting.

Chapter 8: Nutrition and Intermittent Fasting

8.1. Dietary Advice and Recipe Tips for Intermittent Fasting

A crucial component of success in intermittent fasting is adopting a dietary strategy that not only supports the fasting regime but also provides the body with all the necessary nutrients. This section offers practical advice and recipe suggestions to optimize nutrition during eating windows.

Nutritional Planning for Intermittent Fasting

Balancing Macronutrients

During eating windows, it's important to balance macronutrients: proteins, fats, and carbohydrates. Each meal should include a source of lean protein, a moderate portion of complex carbohydrates, and healthy fats.

Nutrient-Dense Foods

Incorporate nutrient-dense foods like leafy green vegetables, fresh fruits, seeds, nuts, legumes, and whole grains. These foods provide vitamins, minerals, fibers, and other health-benefiting compounds.

Meal and Recipe Ideas

Satisfying yet Light Meals

To avoid overeating, prepare meals that are filling but not overly heavy. For example, a quinoa bowl with grilled vegetables, avocado, and a lean protein source like chicken or tofu.

Nutritious Snacks

Prepare nutritious snacks for moments when you feel hungry between meals. Options might include vegetable sticks with hummus, fresh fruit with a handful of nuts, or Greek yogurt with berries.

Importance of Hydration

Recommended Beverages

Maintain adequate hydration by drinking water, unsweetened tea, or herbal infusions. These beverages can help manage hunger and improve metabolism.

Avoid Sugary Drinks

Limit or avoid sugary drinks and alcoholic beverages, which can provide empty calories and negatively impact weight loss efforts.

Adapting Recipes to Individual Preferences

Variation and Creativity

Don't hesitate to vary recipes based on your taste preferences and nutritional needs. Experimenting in the kitchen can make eating during fasting more enjoyable and less repetitive.

Diet and Allergy Considerations

Adapt recipes to meet any dietary restrictions or allergies. There are many alternatives available to adjust meals for vegetarian, vegan, gluten-free, or other specific needs.

Conclusion and Transition to the Next Section

By adopting these dietary tips and experimenting with nutritious recipes, it's possible to make intermittent fasting a delicious and healthy experience. In the next section, we'll explore how to incorporate intermittent fasting into special occasions and holidays, ensuring flexibility and enjoyment without compromising progress.

8.2. Incorporating Intermittent Fasting into Special Occasions and Holidays

Holidays and special occasions can pose unique challenges for those practicing intermittent fasting. However, with planning and flexibility, it's possible to enjoy these times without compromising the benefits of fasting.

Planning and Flexibility

Adjusting Your Fasting Schedule

Consider adjusting your fasting schedule in anticipation of special events. For instance, you might shift your eating windows to align with an event or choose to take a break from fasting for that day.

Anticipate and Plan

If you know a celebration or event is approaching, plan ahead. This might mean being more stringent with fasting in the days leading up to the event or scheduling extra physical exercise.

Enjoying the Event Without Excess

Moderation and Balance

During the event, try to maintain a moderation approach. Enjoy the food and beverages offered but aim to make balanced choices and listen to your body's satiety signals.

Opting for Nutrient-Rich Foods

When possible, lean towards healthier or nutrient-rich options. For example, favor vegetables, salads, lean proteins, and limit high-calorie or sugary foods.

Managing Social Pressures

Explaining Your Approach

If you feel comfortable, explain your intermittent fasting approach to your friends and family. Many people will be understanding and might even be curious or interested.

Feeling No Obligation

Remember, you're not obligated to eat or drink something just because it's offered. Staying true to your health and wellness goals is important.

Post-Event

Gradually Returning to Your Fasting Regime

After an event or celebration, gradually return to your normal fasting regime. Avoid "punishing" yourself with extra-long fasts or severe restrictions.

Evaluation and Learning

Use the experience to assess what worked and what didn't. This can help you better manage similar situations in the future.

Conclusion and Transition to the Next Section

With thoughtful planning and a flexible approach, it's possible to integrate intermittent fasting into special occasions and holidays, enjoying the event without compromising your progress in wellness. In the next section, we'll focus on how to continue evolving and adapting in your intermittent fasting journey, exploring new strategies and adjustments.

8.3. Continuing to Evolve and Adapt in the Intermittent Fasting Journey

The journey of intermittent fasting is not static; it requires ongoing adjustments and evolution to remain effective and sustainable in the long term. The ability to adapt and evolve can ensure that intermittent fasting continues to be a healthy and satisfying approach.

Reevaluation and Adaptation of the Fasting Plan

Listening to Your Body

Regularly take the time to listen to your body and assess how you feel with your current fasting regime. This may include monitoring energy levels, sleep quality, weight, and overall well-being.

Reassessing Goals

Over time, your health and wellness goals may change. Periodically reassess your goals to ensure your fasting regime is still aligned with them.

Experimentation and Flexibility

Trying Different Fasting Methods

Being open to experimenting with different fasting methods can help find what works best for you at different times in your life.

Adaptability to Life Circumstances

Be ready to adjust your fasting regime to changing life circumstances, such as shifts in work routine, family situation, or physical activity level.

Integration with Other Health Practices

Pairing with Other Wellness Aspects

Consider how intermittent fasting can be paired with other healthy practices, such as exercise, meditation, or mindfulness, to maximize overall health benefits.

Consultation with Health Professionals

As you adapt and evolve your fasting regime, consulting health professionals, like nutritionists or doctors, can ensure the changes are safe and effective.

Continuous Learning

Research and Education

Stay informed about the latest research and trends in intermittent fasting. Reading articles, attending webinars, and talking with experts can provide new ideas and inspiration.

Sharing Experiences

Sharing your experiences with others practicing intermittent fasting can offer new perspectives and helpful suggestions.

Maintaining Motivation

Celebrating Successes

Recognize and celebrate your successes along the way. This can include improvements in health, achievement of weight goals, or simply consistency in maintaining the fasting regime.

Setting New Goals

As you adapt and evolve, set new goals to maintain motivation. These can relate to health, fitness, or personal well-being.

Conclusion and Transition to the Next Section

Continually adapting and evolving your approach to intermittent fasting is essential for long-term success. In the next section, we'll explore strategies for overcoming specific obstacles and setbacks that may arise during intermittent fasting.

8.4. Overcoming Obstacles and Setbacks in Intermittent Fasting

Addressing and overcoming obstacles and setbacks is a crucial aspect of maintaining long-term success in intermittent fasting. Understanding how to manage these moments can help keep you on track towards your health and wellness goals.

Identifying Obstacles

Recognizing Challenges

The first step in overcoming obstacles is recognizing them. These can include weight loss plateaus, increased appetite or hunger, or difficulties in maintaining fasting windows.

Analyzing Causes

Once obstacles are identified, it's important to analyze their potential causes. This could relate to lifestyle, eating habits, stress, sleep, or other environmental factors.

Management Strategies

Modifying the Fasting Regime

If a particular fasting schedule is no longer working, consider modifying it. This could mean changing the fasting hours, trying a different fasting method, or incorporating more flexible fasting periods.

Nutritional Balancing

Ensure your nutrition during eating windows is nutritious and balanced. Sometimes, adjusting the proportions of macronutrients or increasing the intake of fiber-rich foods can help overcome a weight loss plateau.

Addressing Emotional Setbacks

Recognizing Emotional Impact

Setbacks can have a significant impact on morale and self-efficacy. Recognizing and addressing emotional responses to these challenges is crucial for recovery and progress.

Coping Strategies

Use positive coping strategies like meditation, physical activity, or sharing your experiences with others to manage negative emotions related to setbacks.

Maintaining a Long-Term Perspective

Holistic View

Maintain a holistic view of your wellness journey. Obstacles and setbacks are natural and part of the journey. Remember that progress is not always linear.

Reevaluation and Setting New Goals

Sometimes, it may be necessary to reevaluate and set new goals that are more aligned with your current circumstances and capabilities.

Seeking Support

Professional Support

Do not hesitate to seek the support of a health professional if you continue to encounter obstacles. A nutritionist, doctor, or coach can provide personalized guidance.

Social Support Network

Lean on your social support network for advice, encouragement, and motivation. Sometimes, sharing your challenges can lighten the emotional load and open new perspectives.

Conclusion and Transition to the Next Section

Overcoming obstacles and setbacks requires patience, flexibility, and an open mind. In the next section, we'll explore the summary and additional resources that can support you on your intermittent fasting journey.

8.5. Summary and Additional Resources for Intermittent Fasting

After exploring various aspects of intermittent fasting, it's useful to summarize the key points and provide additional resources for those who wish to deepen their understanding and practice.

Key Points Summary

Fundamental Principles of Intermittent Fasting

- Intermittent fasting involves alternating periods of eating and fasting.

- Various fasting methods can be adapted to individual needs.

Health and Weight Loss Benefits

- Intermittent fasting can aid in weight loss, improve insulin sensitivity, and support overall health.

Managing Challenges and Obstacles

- Recognizing and overcoming common obstacles is crucial for long-term success.

Importance of Balance and Adaptability

- A balanced and flexible approach is essential to keep intermittent fasting sustainable and beneficial.

Additional Resources

Books and Publications

- Numerous books cover various aspects of intermittent fasting, from basic science to practical strategies.

- Academic publications and research articles can offer evidence-based insights.

Websites and Blogs

- Many websites and blogs are dedicated to intermittent fasting, offering advice, recipes, and success stories.

- Online forums can be a source of support and experience sharing.

Apps and Online Tools

- There are apps to help monitor fasting periods and eating windows.

- Some apps also offer food diaries and nutritional advice.

Support Groups and Communities

- Support groups, both online and in-person, can offer advice, motivation, and a sense of community.

- Participation in groups can also help stay up to date on the latest trends and research.

Continuing Education and Adaptation

Continuous Learning

- The field of intermittent fasting is continuously evolving; staying informed on the latest research and strategies is crucial.

Personal Adaptation

- Continue to adapt and personalize your approach to intermittent fasting based on your experience, lifestyle changes, and goals.

Conclusion and Transition to the Next Section

In conclusion, intermittent fasting is a dynamic journey that requires a consistent commitment to learning, adapting, and personal growth. In the next chapter, we'll begin exploring the first of the specific intermittent fasting methods, providing a detailed guide on how to start and sustain each of them.

Chapter 9: Recipes and Dietary Tips

9.1 Introduction to the 16/8 Method: A Guide and Tips

The 16/8 method is one of the most popular approaches to intermittent fasting. It involves a fasting window of 16 hours followed by an eating window of 8 hours. This chapter provides a detailed guide to getting started with the 16/8 method, offering practical tips for effective practice.

What Is the 16/8 Method

Basic Principles

The 16/8 method entails fasting for 16 consecutive hours and eating during an 8-hour interval.

This pattern can be easily adapted to one's daily routine, choosing the most convenient eating interval.

Benefits

The 16/8 method is known for its simplicity and ease of integration into everyday life.

It's effective for weight loss, improving insulin sensitivity, and may have benefits for overall metabolic health.

How to Start with the 16/8 Method

Choosing Eating Windows

Select an eight-hour interval that fits best into your daily routine. Common eating windows include 12:00-20:00 or 10:00-18:00.

Ensure that the eating interval aligns with your lifestyle, social commitments, and work schedule.

Gradual Introduction

If you're new to intermittent fasting, consider starting gradually by shortening the eating window instead of jumping straight into 16 hours of fasting.

Begin with, for example, 12 hours of fasting and gradually increase to reach 16 hours.

Tips for Managing Fasting

Managing Hunger

Drinking plenty of water during the fasting period can help manage hunger.

Beverages like black tea, green tea, or unsweetened coffee are also allowed and can help suppress appetite.

Physical Activity

Experiment with exercising during the fasting or eating window to see what works best for you.

Some people find benefits in exercising while fasting, while others prefer to work out after eating.

Nutrition during Eating Windows

Focus on Food Quality

During the eating windows, focus on nutritious and balanced foods.

Include a variety of fruits and vegetables, lean proteins, healthy fats, and complex carbohydrates.

Avoid Overeating

Avoid overeating during the eating windows. Listen to your body's satiety signals and avoid eating out of boredom or habit.

Adaptation and Flexibility

Listening to Your Body

Pay close attention to how your body responds to the 16/8 fasting and be willing to make adjustments if necessary.

If you encounter difficulties or discomfort, consider adapting the fasting window or consulting a health professional.

Flexibility for Special Occasions

For special occasions or social events, you may choose to temporarily adjust your fasting schedule.

Conclusion and Transition to the Next Point

The 16/8 method offers a flexible and manageable approach to intermittent fasting, suitable for many lifestyles. In the next section, we will explore another popular intermittent fasting method, the 5:2 method, providing tips and guidelines for its successful implementation.

9.2 Introduction to the 5:2 Method: A Guide and Tips

The 5:2 method is another popular approach to intermittent fasting. Unlike the 16/8 method, the 5:2 involves consuming a very low number of calories for two days a week, while eating normally on the other five days. This chapter offers a detailed guide on how to effectively implement the 5:2 method.

Principles of the 5:2 Method

Fasting Structure

In the 5:2 method, for two non-consecutive days a week, calorie intake is drastically reduced, typically to about 500-600 calories per day.

For the remaining five days, normal eating is resumed without specific caloric restrictions.

Benefits

This method is often preferred by those who find complete fasting or limiting eating windows every day challenging.

It can be effective for weight loss, improving health biomarkers, and increasing longevity.

How to Start with the 5:2 Method

Choosing Fasting Days

Select two days a week that best fit your lifestyle and commitments for your fasting days. Ensure these days are not consecutive to avoid excessive stress on the body.

Planning Low-Calorie Meals

Plan your meals for fasting days in advance, focusing on nutrient-dense, low-calorie foods such as vegetables, fruits, lean proteins, and whole grains.

Tips for Managing Fasting

Managing Hunger

During fasting days, it's normal to experience more hunger than usual. Drinking plenty of water, unsweetened tea, or vegetable broth can help manage hunger sensations.

Light Physical Activity

On fasting days, it might be preferable to opt for light physical activities such as walking or yoga, rather than intense workouts.

Nutritional Strategies

Balance on Non-Fasting Days

On non-fasting days, it's important to maintain a balanced diet and not use these days as an excuse for excessive consumption of unhealthy foods.

Listening to Your Body

Listen to how your body reacts to this fasting pattern and adjust accordingly. If you feel excessively tired or irritable, it might be necessary to review your plan.

Overcoming Common Challenges

Avoiding Overcompensation

Avoid overcompensating on non-fasting days. This can negate the benefits of fasting days.

Support and Motivation

Seek support from friends, family, or online groups to share experiences and stay motivated.

Conclusion and Transition to the Next Point

The 5:2 method offers a flexible approach to intermittent fasting, suitable for those who prefer to limit calorie intake rather than eating windows. In the next section, we will discuss another intermittent fasting method, alternate day fasting, exploring how it can be integrated into your routine.

9.3 Introduction to Alternate-Day Fasting: A Guide and Tips

Alternate-day fasting is another popular approach within intermittent fasting. This method involves alternating days of complete fasting or consuming a very low number of calories, with days where eating is normal. This section offers a detailed guide on how to successfully implement alternate-day fasting.

Principles of Alternate-Day Fasting

Fasting Structure

In this method, fasting days (with no food or an extremely reduced calorie intake, typically around 500 calories) alternate with days where there are no dietary restrictions.

Potential Benefits

Alternate day fasting can be effective for weight loss, improving insulin sensitivity, and potentially offering benefits for heart health and longevity.

Starting with Alternate-Day Fasting

Choosing Fasting Days

Decide which days of the week you will dedicate to fasting. It's important that these days fit well with your lifestyle and commitments.

Preparing for Fasting Days

On fasting days, plan in advance whether you will consume a small number of calories or fast completely. Prepare low-calorie meals or snacks that are nutritious and filling.

Managing Alternate-Day Fasting

Dealing with Hunger

During fasting days, hydration is key. Drink plenty of water, unsweetened tea, or vegetable broth to help manage hunger.

Physical Activity

On fasting days, you might feel less energetic for intense exercises. Listen to your body and adjust the intensity of physical activity accordingly.

Nutrition on Non-Fasting Days

Maintaining a Balanced Diet

On non-fasting days, it's important not to overdo it. Maintain a balanced diet rich in fruits, vegetables, lean proteins, healthy fats, and complex carbohydrates.

Avoiding Excess

Avoid the mindset of "making up for" fasting by overeating on non-fasting days.

Psychological Considerations

Mental Management

Alternate day fasting can be a challenge both physically and mentally. Find strategies to manage cravings and hunger, such as distracting yourself or engaging in enjoyable activities.

Social Support

Having the support of friends, family, or an online community can help stay motivated and committed to the regimen.

Conclusion and Transition to the Next Point

Alternate day fasting offers a diversified approach to intermittent fasting, suitable for those looking for a flexible yet structured strategy. In the next section, we will explore how to assess and monitor progress in intermittent fasting, to ensure it remains a healthy and satisfying journey.

9.4 Assessing and Monitoring Progress in Intermittent Fasting

Tracking and evaluating progress are crucial components for the long-term success of intermittent fasting. Being aware of physical, emotional, and lifestyle changes can help make necessary adjustments and maintain motivation.

Importance of Monitoring

Objective Evaluation

Monitoring progress through objective measures such as weight, body measurements, or energy levels can provide concrete feedback on performance and outcomes.

Recognizing Changes

Noticing changes in sleep, mood, concentration, and overall health can indicate the positive or negative impact of intermittent fasting on your life.

Monitoring Tools

Food and Activity Journals

Keeping a food or activity journal can help track what you eat and how much you move, offering a clear view of your daily behaviors.

Apps and Tracking Devices

Using smartphone apps or wearable devices can provide a simple and automatic way to track physical activity, calorie intake, and fasting progress.

Listening to Your Body

Physical Sensations and Hunger

Pay attention to how you feel during fasting and eating periods. If you experience negative symptoms such as excessive fatigue, irritability, or difficulty concentrating, it may be necessary to review your fasting regimen.

Adjustments Based on Personal Feedback

Use your body's feedback to make adjustments in your fasting regimen. This could include changing the duration of fasting, the frequency, or the composition of meals.

General Health Assessment

Regular Medical Check-ups

Regular medical visits and check-ups can help monitor the impact of intermittent fasting on your overall health and identify any areas of concern.

Monitoring Biomarkers

Monitoring biomarkers such as blood sugar, cholesterol, and blood pressure can provide valuable insights into the physical benefits of intermittent fasting.

Setting and Achieving Goals

Short and Long-Term Goals

Setting clear, both short and long-term, goals can help maintain direction and motivation in your fasting journey.

Celebrating Successes

Celebrating milestones, even small progresses, can strengthen motivation and provide a sense of achievement.

Conclusion and Transition to the Next Section

Assessing and monitoring progress in intermittent fasting is essential to keep the journey effective and rewarding. In the next section, we will focus on how to manage and adapt intermittent fasting during periods of stress and life changes, to ensure the practice remains sustainable.

9.5 Managing and Adapting Intermittent Fasting During Periods of Stress and Life Changes

Life is full of changes and challenges, including periods of high stress. During these times, it may be necessary to adapt your intermittent fasting practice to ensure it remains beneficial and sustainable.

Recognizing the Impact of Stress

Effects of Stress on the Body

Stress can significantly impact metabolism, appetite, and energy levels, affecting the ability to maintain an effective fasting regime.

Listening to Body Signals

During periods of high stress, listen carefully to your body. You may need more energy or nutrients, or you might find it more challenging to stick to a strict fasting schedule.

Adapting the Fasting Regimen

Flexibility in Fasting

Consider adapting your fasting regimen to make it more manageable. This might mean shortening fasting windows or reducing the frequency of fasting days.

Priority on Nutrition

Ensure your meals are particularly nutritious and balanced during times of stress. Focus on foods that provide sustained energy and help manage stress, such as those rich in omega-3s, magnesium, and vitamin B.

Stress Management

Stress-Reduction Techniques

Implement stress-reduction techniques such as meditation, regular exercise, or spending time in nature to help better manage stress.

Emotional Aspects

Acknowledge and address the emotional aspects of stress. Sometimes, stress can lead to emotional eating, which can interfere with intermittent fasting.

Support During Life Changes

Consultation with Health Professionals

During significant life changes, such as pregnancy, a job change, or illness, it's important to consult a health professional to assess how best to adapt intermittent fasting.

Seeking Support

Don't hesitate to seek emotional and practical support from friends, family, or support groups.

Periodic Reevaluation

Monitoring Changes

Monitor how life changes affect your overall well-being and your ability to maintain intermittent fasting.

Adjustments Based on Self-Assessment

Be prepared to make adjustments in your fasting regimen based on your self-assessment and body feedback.

Conclusion and Transition to the Next Section

Managing and adapting intermittent fasting during periods of stress and life changes is crucial to ensure the practice remains beneficial and sustainable. In the next chapter, we will begin to explore intermittent fasting and physical activity, examining how to effectively balance these two important aspects of well-being.

Chapter 10: Summary and Final Reflections

10.1 Intermittent Fasting and Physical Activity: Balancing Exercise and Nutrition

Incorporating physical activity into intermittent fasting requires careful balancing to maximize the benefits of both exercise and fasting. This chapter explores how to effectively synchronize nutrition and exercise within the context of intermittent fasting.

Understanding the Interaction Between Fasting and Exercise

Effects of Fasting on Exercise

Fasting can impact your energy and performance during exercise. Some people experience increased energy and mental clarity, while others may feel more tired.

Benefits of Exercising in a Fasted State

Exercising in a fasted state can potentially enhance lipolysis (fat burning) and improve metabolic adaptability. However, the response varies from individual to individual.

Strategies for Balancing Fasting and Exercise

Planning Exercise Around Eating Windows

For some, exercising just before the eating window can be effective, allowing the body to be nourished right after exercise.

Experimenting with Timing

Others may find it more effective to exercise during the fasting window. It's important to experiment to find what works best for you.

Listening to Your Body

Pay close attention to how you feel during and after exercising in relation to your fasting. Adjust the intensity and duration of exercise based on your energy and strength levels.

Nutrition and Recovery

Importance of Post-Exercise Nutrition

Ensure you consume nutritious meals after exercising, especially if you work out towards the end of your fasting period. These meals should include a good mix of proteins, carbohydrates, and healthy fats to aid in recovery.

Hydration

Maintaining proper hydration is vital, especially if you exercise in a fasted state. Water, naturally flavored water, and herbal teas are excellent options.

Types of Exercise and Intermittent Fasting

Exercise Variation

Vary the type of physical activity. Activities like yoga, pilates, and walking can be more manageable on fasting days, while high-intensity workouts can be scheduled for non-fasting days.

Listening to Fatigue Signals

If you feel excessively tired or unable to perform at your usual level, it could be a sign that your body needs more nutrition or a change in your fasting regimen.

Conclusion and Transition to the Next Section

Balancing physical activity with intermittent fasting requires experimentation and listening to your body. In the next section, we will focus on how intermittent fasting can be customized based on various lifestyles and individual needs.

10.2 Customizing Intermittent Fasting Based on Lifestyle and Individual Needs

The long-term success of intermittent fasting largely depends on its adaptability to individual needs, lifestyles, and preferences. This section explores how to personalize intermittent fasting to make it more effective and sustainable.

Understanding Your Needs

Assessment of Living Conditions

Consider factors like your work schedule, family commitments, social activities, and stress levels when choosing a fasting method. Fasting should fit seamlessly into your daily routine, not hinder it.

Listening to Your Body

Observe how you physically and emotionally respond to fasting. Some may tolerate prolonged fasting well, while others might need more frequent or longer eating windows.

Adapting the Fasting Method

Choosing the Appropriate Method

Among methods such as 16/8, 5:2, or alternate day fasting, choose the one that best suits your lifestyle and nutritional needs.

Flexibility in the Regimen

Be ready to modify your fasting regimen according to changes in your life. Flexibility can help keep fasting sustainable in the long term.

Balancing with Nutrition

Adapting Nutrition

Your nutrition on non-fasting days or during eating windows should compensate for nutritional needs. This includes adequate intake of macro and micronutrients.

Special Considerations for Specific Diets

For those following special diets, like vegan, vegetarian, or gluten-free, it's essential to ensure fasting doesn't lead to nutritional deficiencies.

Managing Social and Work Commitments

Social Planning

Adapt your fasting to social commitments. For example, you might choose to shift fasting windows or take a break from fasting for special events.

Work-Life Balance

If your job requires high mental or physical energy, ensure your fasting regimen does not compromise your work capacity.

Listening and Acting on Feedback

Periodic Reevaluation

Regularly review the effectiveness of your fasting regime. Feel free to experiment and change approaches until you find what works best for you.

Monitoring Health and Well-being

Continue to monitor your overall health and well-being to ensure fasting is having a positive impact.

Conclusion and Transition to the Next Section

Customizing intermittent fasting based on personal needs and lifestyles is crucial to maintaining the practice as rewarding and effective. In the next section, we will discuss strategies for incorporating intermittent fasting sustainably over the long term.

10.3 Incorporating Intermittent Fasting in a Sustainable Way Long-Term

Long-term sustainability is a key factor for the continued success of intermittent fasting. This section explores how to maintain intermittent fasting as a sustainable and beneficial part of your lifestyle over the long term.

Establishing a Sustainable Routine

Adapting to Daily Life

Find a balance that allows fasting to integrate into your daily life without causing undue stress or inconvenience. Long-term sustainability requires the fasting to adapt to your routine, not the other way around.

Avoiding Excessive Rigidity

Avoid being too rigid in your fasting regime. Allow yourself some flexibility for social events, stressful days, or when you simply don't feel at your best.

Listening and Responding to Your Body

Physical and Emotional Signals

Pay attention to your body's signals. If you start feeling tired, irritable, or notice other negative changes, it may be necessary to reconsider your approach to fasting.

Adjustments Based on Needs

Be willing to make adjustments based on how you feel. This might mean changing the frequency, duration, or type of intermittent fasting you are practicing.

Maintaining Nutritional Balance

Importance of Nutrition

During eating windows, focus on the quality of food. A balanced diet, rich in essential nutrients, is crucial to maintain health and energy.

Avoiding Compensation with Food

Do not use eating windows as an opportunity for excessive consumption or to eat unhealthy foods in large quantities. Maintain a healthy balance.

Support and Community

Support Network

Having a support network, whether it's friends, family, or online groups, can provide extra encouragement and a place to share experiences and advice.

Sharing Experiences

Sharing your experience with intermittent fasting can be motivating and informative, both for you and others.

Regular Review and Adjustment

Regular Evaluation

Take time to regularly assess your experience with intermittent fasting. This includes reviewing your progress, how you feel physically and emotionally, and how fasting is impacting your life.

Adjustments Based on Outcomes

Be ready to make adjustments based on the outcomes of your assessment. This might mean changing your fasting regime or making changes to your diet and lifestyle.

Conclusion and Transition to the Next Section

Maintaining intermittent fasting sustainably over the long term requires balance, flexibility, and attentive listening to your own body and needs. In the next section, we will explore the role of health professionals in supporting your intermittent fasting journey.

10.4 The Role of Health Professionals in Supporting Intermittent Fasting

The involvement of health professionals can play a crucial role in ensuring that intermittent fasting is practiced safely and effectively. This chapter explores how health professionals can assist in your intermittent fasting journey.

Preventive Consultation

Health Assessment

Before starting intermittent fasting, it's advisable to consult a doctor, especially if you have pre-existing medical conditions or are taking medication.

Personalized Plans

Health professionals can help develop a fasting plan that considers your specific health needs, goals, and lifestyle.

Health Monitoring

Regular Check-ups

Regular check-ups can monitor the effects of fasting on your general health, including parameters like weight, cholesterol levels, and blood pressure.

Identification of Possible Issues

A health professional can quickly identify any health issues that may arise as a result of fasting and advise appropriate adjustments.

Nutritional Support

Advice from Nutritionists

A nutritionist can provide valuable guidance on meal composition during eating windows, ensuring you receive adequate nutrition.

Dietary Adjustments

Nutrition professionals can help adapt your diet to manage or prevent issues such as nutrient deficiencies or metabolic imbalances.

Management of Specific Medical Conditions

Personalized Strategies

For conditions such as diabetes, heart problems, or eating disorders, a personalized approach to fasting is essential.

Monitoring of Existing Conditions

Monitoring how fasting affects any existing medical condition is vital to ensure it doesn't compromise your overall health.

Psychological Aspects of Fasting

Psychological Support

Mental health professionals can offer support for any emotional or psychological issues that may arise from fasting, such as food anxiety or obsession with food and weight.

Coping Strategies

Involvement of a therapist can be helpful in providing strategies to manage stress or any other emotional challenges related to fasting.

Involvement in the Long-Term Journey

Ongoing Support

Regular communication with health professionals can provide ongoing support, allowing for adjustments and optimizations over time.

Periodic Evaluation of Outcomes

Health professionals can help periodically assess the outcomes of fasting, ensuring your health and well-being goals are achieved.

Conclusion and Transition to the Next Section

The involvement of health professionals is crucial to ensure that intermittent fasting is practiced in a safe and personalized manner. In the next section, we will explore how to address and overcome common myths and misunderstandings about intermittent fasting.

10.5 Addressing and Overcoming Myths and Misconceptions About Intermittent Fasting

Intermittent fasting is often surrounded by myths and misconceptions that can create confusion and hinder effective practice. This chapter aims to clarify these misunderstandings and provide evidence-based information.

Myth 1: Fasting Causes Muscle Loss

Reality

Although weight loss may include some loss of muscle mass, intermittent fasting, when combined with a balanced diet and regular physical activity, does not necessarily cause significant muscle loss.

Studies suggest that intermittent fasting may actually enhance muscle preservation compared to traditional calorie-restriction diets.

Myth 2: Fasting Puts the Body into 'Starvation Mode'

Reality

"Starvation mode," or a significant reduction in metabolism, is generally a concern only in cases of extreme caloric restriction or prolonged fasting.

Intermittent fasting, practiced in a balanced way, does not push the body into this mode; in fact, it can increase metabolism in the short term.

Myth 3: Fasting is Dangerous and Unhealthy

Reality

When done correctly and in the absence of pre-existing medical conditions that contraindicate it, intermittent fasting is generally safe and can offer health benefits.

However, it's important to start gradually and, if necessary, under the supervision of a health professional.

Myth 4: Fasting Means Eating Nothing

Reality

Intermittent fasting does not necessarily mean eating nothing for extended periods. It depends on the chosen method; some forms of intermittent fasting allow for very low-calorie consumption, while others are based on alternating between fasting and eating windows.

Myth 5: Fasting is Suitable for Everyone

Reality

Intermittent fasting may not be suitable for everyone. Individuals with certain health conditions, pregnant or breastfeeding women, and those with a history of eating disorders should avoid intermittent fasting or proceed only with caution and under medical supervision.

Myth 6: Fasting Is the Only Solution for Weight Loss

Reality

While intermittent fasting can be an effective method for weight loss for some people, it is not the only solution. A balanced diet and regular physical activity are fundamental components of a healthy weight loss regime.

Conclusion and Transition to the Next Section

Addressing and overcoming these myths is crucial for an accurate understanding and effective practice of intermittent fasting. In the next section, we will discuss how to incorporate intermittent fasting into a comprehensive wellness plan.

Chapter 11: Additional Resources and Conclusion

11.1 Incorporating Intermittent Fasting into a Comprehensive Wellness Plan

The effectiveness of intermittent fasting is amplified when it is part of a comprehensive wellness plan that embraces all aspects of health and well-being. This section explores how to integrate intermittent fasting into a holistic approach to health.

Creating a Holistic Balance

Beyond Weight Control

Consider intermittent fasting as one tool among many in a holistic approach to health, which includes a balanced diet, physical exercise, adequate sleep, and stress management.

Integration with Diet

Ensure your diet provides a variety of essential nutrients. Intermittent fasting is not an excuse for a poor diet on non-fasting days.

Physical Exercise and Intermittent Fasting

Combining with Physical Activity

Synchronize your exercise regime with your fasting schedule. For example, some find it beneficial to exercise at the end of their fasting period to maximize fat burning.

Variation and Moderation

Vary your workouts to include both cardio and strength exercises, and adjust the intensity based on your fasting and eating windows.

Stress Management and Recovery

Stress-Reduction Techniques

Incorporate practices such as yoga, meditation, or walks in nature to reduce stress, which can significantly impact health and the success of intermittent fasting.

Importance of Sleep

Prioritize quality sleep, as lack of sleep can negatively affect hunger, appetite, and metabolism.

Monitoring and Adapting

Listening to the Body

Be attentive to your body's signals and adapt your fasting practice, diet, and exercise based on how you feel.

Periodic Reviews

Conduct periodic reviews of your wellness approach to ensure intermittent fasting integrates well with other aspects of your health.

Support and Community

Seeking Support

Do not hesitate to seek support from health professionals, friends, and online communities that can offer advice, encouragement, and new perspectives.

Sharing and Learning

Share your experience with others and remain open to learning from others' stories and advice.

Conclusion and Transition to the Next Section

Incorporating intermittent fasting into a comprehensive wellness plan can lead to significant improvements in physical and mental health. In the next section, we will explore success stories and testimonials to provide further motivation and perspectives on intermittent fasting.

11.2 Success Stories and Testimonials on Intermittent Fasting

Success stories can be a source of inspiration and learning, offering real-life perspectives on the effectiveness of intermittent fasting. This chapter compiles testimonials and stories from individuals who have experienced transformative effects with intermittent fasting.

Diversity of Experiences

Wide Spectrum of Stories

Testimonials include people of various ages, genders, and backgrounds sharing their experiences with different methods of intermittent fasting.

Unique Outcomes

Each story highlights how intermittent fasting has uniquely impacted weight loss, mental health, energy, physical health, and overall well-being.

Physical Transformation Stories

Weight Loss and Body Composition

Many individuals share how intermittent fasting has aided in their weight loss and improved body composition, often after years of struggling with traditional diets.

Improvements in Physical Health

Some recount improvements in cholesterol levels, blood pressure, insulin sensitivity, and reduction of symptoms of conditions like type 2 diabetes.

Impacts on Mental Health and Well-being

Mental Clarity and Energy

Many report an increase in mental clarity and energy levels, attributing to intermittent fasting a role in their enhanced focus and productivity.

Relationship with Food

Testimonies often include stories about how intermittent fasting has improved people's relationship with food, helping them develop healthier and more mindful eating habits.

Challenges and How They Were Overcome

Addressing Initial Difficulties

Stories include the initial challenges, such as managing hunger, changing eating habits, and integrating fasting into social and family life.

Adaptation Strategies

Strategies adopted to overcome these difficulties are shared, such as meal planning, support from friends and family, and attentive listening to one's body.

Conclusions and Personal Reflections

Lessons and Growth

Testimonials often reflect on what individuals have learned from these experiences, including personal growth and a new understanding of health and well-being.

Advice for Others

Many stories include advice for others who are considering or starting intermittent fasting, providing practical tips based on real-life experiences.

Conclusion and Transition to the Next Section

These success stories offer an authentic and motivating view of intermittent fasting, showcasing a range of paths and possible outcomes. In the next section, we will discuss how to maintain and continue to build on these successes over time.

11.3 Maintaining and Building on the Successes of Intermittent Fasting Long-Term

Maintaining the benefits of intermittent fasting requires ongoing commitment and strategies to build on the achievements already made. This section explores how to sustain and further improve the results of intermittent fasting over time.

Continuous Evaluation

Regular Monitoring

Continue to monitor key aspects of your health and well-being, such as weight, body composition, energy levels, and mental state. This helps to maintain awareness and make any necessary adjustments.

Listening to Your Body

Stay attuned to the signals your body sends you. If you start feeling less energetic or notice other changes, it might be time to review your approach to fasting.

Developing Sustainable Habits

Integration into Daily Life

Find ways to make intermittent fasting a natural and manageable part of your daily routine. This can include adapting fasting windows to fit your schedule or developing healthy eating habits during non-fasting periods.

Flexibility and Adaptability

Be flexible and ready to adjust your fasting regime based on life changes, such as variations in your routine, work commitments, or family obligations.

Strengthening Overall Health

Balanced and Nutritious Diet

Ensure to maintain a rich and varied diet that provides all the necessary nutrients to support your lifestyle and health goals.

Regular Physical Activity

Incorporate regular physical exercise into your lifestyle. Physical activity not only supports weight loss and overall health but can also enhance the effectiveness of intermittent fasting.

Stress Management and Recovery

Stress-Reduction Techniques

Continue to use or develop stress-reduction techniques such as meditation, yoga, or relaxing hobbies, which can help manage stress and improve sleep quality.

Prioritizing Sleep

Maintain a regular and quality sleep routine. Adequate sleep is crucial for weight management, metabolism, and overall health.

Continuous Development and Learning

Research and Education

Stay informed about the latest research and best practices in the field of intermittent fasting. This can include reading books, articles, or participating in seminars and workshops.

Sharing Experiences

Share your experiences with others. Sharing can offer new perspectives and encouragement, both for you and others in the intermittent fasting community.

Conclusion and Transition to the Next Section

Maintaining the successes achieved with intermittent fasting and building on them requires a well-thought-out strategy and ongoing commitment. In the next section, we will address how to navigate and manage periods of plateau or stall in intermittent fasting.

11.4 Navigating and Managing Plateaus or Stalls in Intermittent Fasting

Even in the journey of intermittent fasting, it's common to encounter periods of plateau or stall, where progress seems to slow down or halt. This section explores strategies to manage and overcome these periods.

Recognizing the Plateau

Identification of Stall Periods

A plateau can manifest in various ways, such as a lack of changes in weight, body measurements, or the general feeling of well-being and health.

Acknowledging that plateaus are a normal part of the weight loss and health improvement process is crucial.

Analyzing Your Regimen

Review of Eating Habits

Review your nutrition during non-fasting windows. Ensure you're not unconsciously compensating for fasting with an increased caloric intake or choosing less healthy foods.

Evaluation of Physical Activity

Consider if your physical exercise routine needs adjustments. Increasing the intensity, duration, or frequency of exercise can help overcome the plateau.

Strategies for Breaking the Plateau

Variation of Fasting Regimen

Experiment with different fasting patterns. Changing the duration of fasting or trying a different method can stimulate new progress.

Improvement of Sleep Quality

Sleep plays a crucial role in regulating metabolism and hormones that affect hunger. Improving sleep quality can help overcome the plateau.

Nutritional and Professional Support

Consultation with a Nutritionist

A nutritionist can provide personalized advice to optimize your diet and ensure you're receiving the necessary nutrients to support your fasting regimen.

Medical Check-Up

In some cases, a plateau may be a sign of other underlying issues. A medical check-up can help rule out or manage any health problems.

Emotional and Mental Management

Dealing with Frustration

Addressing the emotions related to the plateau is important. Recognizing and accepting these feelings can help maintain a positive and constructive perspective.

Coping Strategies

Practices like mindfulness, meditation, or recreational activities can help manage stress and frustration related to stall periods.

Maintaining Motivation

Celebrating Other Types of Progress

Besides weight and body measurements, there are many other health and well-being indicators to celebrate, such as improvements in energy, sleep, or mental health.

Reestablishing Goals

Sometimes, reestablishing or adjusting your goals can provide new motivation and a clear direction forward.

Conclusion and Transition to the Next Section

Periods of plateau or stall in intermittent fasting can be challenging, but with the right strategies, it's possible to navigate them and get back on the path to progress. In the next section, we will discuss the future of intermittent fasting and emerging trends in this field.

11.5 The Future of Intermittent Fasting: Emerging Trends and Innovations

As intermittent fasting continues to gain popularity and attention, new trends and innovations are emerging that could shape its future practice. This section explores the potential directions in which intermittent fasting may evolve and how these could shape personal well-being and public health.

Technological Innovations

Apps and Wearables

The ongoing development of health monitoring apps and wearable devices promises to make fasting tracking more intuitive and informative, providing real-time feedback on various health aspects.

Artificial Intelligence and Personalization

The use of artificial intelligence in digital health could lead to highly personalized fasting programs, tailored to an individual's metabolic needs and health goals.

Scientific and Clinical Research

Research Insights

Continued research is exploring the long-term effects of intermittent fasting on longevity, disease prevention, and mental health.

New Fasting Models

Scientific inquiries may uncover new fasting models based on recent discoveries in the fields of nutrition and physiology.

Integration with Conventional Medicine

Holistic Health Approach

Intermittent fasting could be more closely integrated into conventional medical recommendations as part of a holistic approach to weight management, diabetes control, and disease prevention.

Collaboration with Health Professionals

Collaboration between intermittent fasting experts and healthcare professionals could enhance the efficacy and safety of fasting as a therapeutic tool.

Social and Ethical Challenges

Accessibility and Equity

Addressing the issue of accessibility to information and resources for intermittent fasting is crucial, ensuring that people from various socioeconomic backgrounds can benefit.

Education and Awareness

Increasing education and public awareness about intermittent fasting can help debunk myths and promote a deeper understanding of its benefits and practices.

Evolution of Eating Habits and Lifestyle

Sustainability and Environment

Intermittent fasting could be explored as part of a sustainable lifestyle, with positive implications for individual health and the environment.

Cultural Adaptation

Adapting intermittent fasting to different food cultures and lifestyles can lead to broader acceptance and global integration.

Conclusion

The future of intermittent fasting looks promising, with potential developments in technology, research, integrated medicine, and social awareness. As the practice continues to evolve, staying informed and adaptable to new developments remains important.

Concluding this journey through the world of intermittent fasting, I want to leave you with some reflections that I hope can accompany you on your personal journey.

Intermittent fasting is not just a dietary practice; it's a journey of personal discovery. It's about listening to and understanding your body, experimenting and adapting, and finding a balance that works for you in your unique and precious life. Remember, every small step you take is an act of care for yourself, a commitment to your health and well-being.

There will be moments of challenge, periods of doubt, and times when results seem far away. In these moments, I encourage you to remember why you started this journey. Recall the small victories and the lessons learned along the way. Celebrate every success, no matter how small, and be kind to yourself in tough times.

Intermittent fasting is more than a methodology; it's a journey that reveals the strength of perseverance, the beauty of self-discipline, and the power of awareness. This journey invites you to reconnect with yourself in ways you may not have considered before, opening the door to a new understanding of health, nourishment, and overall well-being.

As you proceed, know that you are not alone on this journey. There is a community of people around the world who share your experiences, your challenges, and your successes. Find strength in their company and inspiration in their stories.

Finally, remember that the journey toward well-being is as important as the destination. Every day is an opportunity to learn something new about yourself and to make choices that reflect your commitment to your health. Be proud of what you have achieved and excited about the possibilities that are yet to come.

I wish you a journey full of discoveries, health, and happiness. May your path with intermittent fasting be enlightening, rewarding, and transformative.

If this book has positively impacted you and been helpful, I would be grateful if you could take a moment to share your impressions with a brief review on Amazon.

Thank you,

Giuliano Monti